AGING
STRONGER

THE ULTIMATE GUIDE TO OVERCOMING PAIN AND INJURY WITHOUT RELYING ON MEDICATIONS, INJECTIONS, OR SURGERY

DR. JACK W. WONG

ACKNOWLEDGEMENTS

To my family:

Kimberly, for supporting me and believing that I can make the world a better place.

Lai Wah, for inspiring me to never give up during times of adversity

Franklin and Kevin, for your unconditional love

To my mentors:

Lloyd Kimerling, for keeping me grounded all these years

Greg Todd, for lighting up my entrepreneurial journey

Paul Gough, for teaching me life and business skills

Anil Gupta, for helping me find my purpose

Dennis Cummins, for helping me share my gift through communication

ABOUT THE AUTHOR

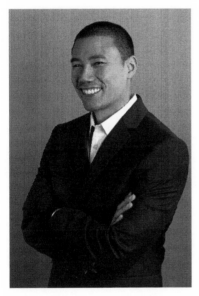

Dr. Jack Wong is a physical therapist and founder of Houston's leading specialist physical therapy company, Next Level Physical Therapy. He specializes in helping people aged 50+ overcome pain and injury using holistic solutions that do not involve medications, injections, or surgery.

Dr. Wong founded Next Level Physical Therapy in 2017 after observing how many clients were not making significant improvements under the traditional western medical system. Since then, he has helped thousands of clients avoid opiate dependency, numerous trips to the doctor's office, and unnecessary surgery. When he isn't treating clients at work, Dr. Wong is playing basketball, lifting weights, or spending time with his beautiful wife, Kimberly.

TESTIMONIALS

"Jack has been my life saver. I've been dealing with a bulging disk. After trying cervical epidurals, oral steroids, chiropractic therapy, and NSAIDs, nothing would help with the burning sensation and pain. Then I finally met Dr. Jack. I didn't have much hope anymore, but I gave him a chance, and it was the best decision I've ever made. He has been able to help me with my symptoms as well as my depression from going through this whole ordeal. He always hears me out and understands me. Best of all, he takes my symptoms away. I love going to my therapy sessions because I know for sure that I will leave pain and stress FREE. Thank you so much, Jack. May god bless you with many years so you can fix many more people."

-Saira

"In my first experience with Dr. Jack Wong, he has really impressed me with his knowledge and professionalism. His attitude is exceptional. He was extremely thorough in finding out what I wanted to achieve as well as problems that I had no idea existed or were possible to improve. In just three sessions, Jack has helped me feel better and provided exercises for continued improvement. He has already improved my balance and corrected a shoulder problem. He also improved my swallowing, which went back to early age tonsillectomy. It took 5 minutes. I heartily recommend Dr. Jack and Next Level Physical Therapy."

-Carl

"Dr. Wong is a very caring practitioner. He's an expert on the mechanics of the anatomy, so he quickly identified my knee problem. He designed a custom workout plan that's really working to ease the pain in my joints. I highly recommend him to anyone who's suffering from chronic joint pain. For me, this is a better option than knee surgery."

-Scott

"I fractured my patella early this year. Having never broken a bone in my body, I was worried about the recovery process. Now I know I had nothing to worry about. My orthopedist said that I am healing faster than most of his patients. I credit this all to Dr. Wong for providing me the tools I needed to succeed. I set small goals for myself, and Dr. Wong's dedication and patience helped me to successfully accomplish them. He is overall a great physical therapist and an even better person."

-Patty

"Jack is hands down the best physical therapist! In several short sessions, I've made more progress on pain, tightness, and scars than years of seeing chiropractors, orthopedic doctors, physical therapists, and surgeons. He utilizes MPS, which is not only unique for scar revision but at the end of each session and for several days after has an overall calming effect. He always explains to you the anatomy behind your issue (or, in my case, issues!) and the reasons why his techniques work. He is truly passionate about what he does, and it shows! Before resorting to medication or surgery, go see Dr. Jack. He will help you get to the root of what's causing your pain and put you on the healing path."

-Jennifer

"Jack is an extremely well-trained and dedicated physical therapist. His approach combines the best of both Western and Asian medical practices. When other practitioners could do nothing for my chronic pain and swelling, Jack was able to remedy the problem within three months. I would unreservedly recommend him for care of patients with chronic conditions. As a physician, I care deeply about what is done to my aging body; Jack is careful, considerate, and a consummate care giver."

-Doc Bob

"My son went to Jack for back and leg pain and found immediate relief after just 1 MPS treatment, something acupuncture could not do. After several more treatments, he is happily back to normal. Now I am seeing Jack for shoulder stiffness, pain, and inflammation from Rheumatoid Arthritis and have noticed significant improvements. Jack is very knowledgeable and courteous and is very driven to help you improve no matter what your condition. I am so grateful for MPS and for Jack helping my body heal itself through cutting edge treatment."

-Joanie

"Jack is the most knowledgeable and hands-on physical therapist I've come across. After 8 years of physical therapy and working with over 20 individuals, I am finally receiving help that is effective. His explanations are clear and easy to follow. I'm thankful to have found Next Level Physical Therapy."

-Lori

"I began going to Next Level Physical Therapy at age 65 after experiencing severe back pain from unknown spinal stenosis. I was unable to stand for more than 10-15 minutes or walk more than 100 yards. Doctors diagnosed me but were unable to treat my condition. I couldn't take anti-inflammatories such as NSAIDs or oral steroids. Spinal steroid injections were ineffective. Prior to my stenosis, I regularly walked 2-3 miles a day.

"I went to therapy twice a week for a few months. Dr. Jack Wong was incredible in his concern, instruction, and all around care for me. We gradually built up the intensity of the exercises. He made sure that I understood the process and could do the exercises at home. Jack insisted that I keep him informed of any problems or successes between my visits, even while he was on vacation.

"I said I hoped to go on my favorite retreat in November, which would require several hours in a car and lots of walking. With Jack's help, I made it to the retreat with some accommodations. After that, I wanted to return to hiking in nature as I loved to do. I am excited to say that I regularly hike at the arboretum and that on my last vacation I hiked 2-4 miles a day for four days in a row. I attribute my success to Dr. Jack Wong and his practice, Next Level Physical Therapy, who gave me my freedom and joy back. Not only is my back issue much improved, but my whole body is stronger than it's ever been. In the process, I have learned valuable lessons to help keep me healthy in my senior years."

-Dan

"Dr. Jack Wong worked wonders for me. I injured my back after we were flooded by Hurricane Harvey. All the lifting reignited an old injury, but it was worse this time. I tried ibuprofen, Tylenol, and exercises I received from a physical therapist years ago. The pain and stiffness would start to get better, but the relief would not last. I kept finding myself right back where I started. After several months, I gave up and decided to seek professional help. I wish I had started with Dr. Wong in the beginning instead of thinking I could do it myself. I wasted a lot of time and prolonged the pain.

"Dr. Wong gave me an evaluation and developed a plan that helped me regain strength and flexibility gradually. He knew what exercises to start with and when we needed to increase the difficulty. When I tried to do that myself, I re-aggravated the injury and never made progress, but I have not had any setbacks while following Dr. Wong's instructions. I can now do things again without injury. I am back to working in the yard, on the cars, and carrying things around the house. I can carry suitcases again and take trips without pain and my previous limitations. I still have to be careful, but he taught me how to do that, what to look out for, and why problems happen. He made a huge difference in the quality of my life, and I appreciate his expertise, his thoroughness, and his professionalism. He was great to work with and produced results, exactly what you hope for in a doctor."

-John

TABLE OF CONTENTS

CHAPTER 1

MINDSET SHIFT

Be comfortable with being uncomfortable.
Be uncomfortable with being comfortable.

When was the last time you took a shortcut even though you knew there was a better alternative? We all do it. We get fast food instead of cooking a healthy meal. We hop on the treadmill rather than doing a full workout. We down a few extra cups of coffee to stay up late when we know we should get some sleep. When we're young, we can get away with it. But as we get older, our bodies change. What worked in the past, whether exercise or diet, may not work anymore. That doesn't mean we're doomed to a life of pain and limitations. It means we have to stop taking shortcuts.

This book was written to let people over 50 know that pain, decreased mobility, and loss of independence are not part of the normal aging process. In it, you'll learn how using natural solutions to treat the cause of your pain instead of the symptoms is the only way to long-term health and wellness. It may be uncomfortable to give up the old shortcuts and adopt new habits, but as Albert Einstein (maybe) once said, "the definition of insanity is doing the same thing over and over and expecting a different result." If the old methods aren't working for you now, I challenge you to try some of the tips in this book. See for yourself the transformation in your health and body.

I started my PT career in an outpatient clinic where I focused mainly on the patient's diagnosis, treating the painful or injured body part. I thought all of my clients wanted to get out of pain and nothing more. Over the years, I realized that people live with pain all the time. They might resort to consuming pain medications for years until they no longer work, only to seek a higher dosage or another type of pain pill. Some just keep adding more and more pills. Polypharmacy is the use of multiple drugs to treat a single condition or the simultaneous use of multiple medications by a single client for one or more conditions. According to the Washington Post, 25 percent of people aged 65 to 69 take at least five prescription drugs, and 46 percent of those are between age 70 and 79.

After my stint in outpatient therapy, I transitioned to home health. In my clients' homes, I saw firsthand the dangers of taking multiple medications. Increased medication consumption is directly correlated to an increase in side effects and overdoses. It wasn't pretty. They were stuck taking medications because they weren't given better alternatives.

When I started my own practice, I wanted to help people do more than just manage their pain with medications. In fact, pain isn't the primary reason people call my clinic; it is the increased difficulty or inability to perform the activity they love doing. Losing something they love wakes them up from the vicious cycle of pain medications, injections, and surgery. Many people who are living with pain are currently stuck, not sure where to go for the right information. They have been let down by their doctors, other healthcare professionals, and the traditional western healthcare model. My hope is that the information in this book will make you aware of an alternative to the traditional medicine model to help you get unstuck and start living a fulfilling life free of pain killers, injections, and unnecessary surgery.

THE POWER OF COMPOUNDING EFFECT

"Compound interest is the eighth wonder of the world. He who understands it, earns it ... he who doesn't ... pays it."

Compounding effect is the same concept in health as in finance: taking small steps will generate immense changes over time. The two major factors at play are consistency of action and time. Think of your normal everyday routine. What kinds of food do you eat and what kinds of activities do you participate in? Over time, those habits have an enormous impact on your health. Time can either be your best friend, if you have good habits, or your worst enemy, if you have bad habits.

How would you rate your overall health right now? What are some areas where you can improve? Making any changes can be scary and uncomfortable, but if you take small steps consistently, most goals are achievable over time. The perfect example is of a baby learning how to walk. Once, you were a baby who was crawling. Then you learned to stand. Finally, after plenty of practice (and falls), you were strong enough to walk.

The power of mindset can also be compounded in a positive or negative way. According to the law of attraction, if you focus on negative ideas, that is what will come your way. The same is true for positive thoughts.

What kind of bad habits can you replace with better habits? What kind of changes would it provide to your life if you were consistent with these good habits? Many of the strategies in this book about solving your pain naturally require small steps over time, which leads to big changes.

LET THE COMPOUND EFFECT WORK FOR YOU

1. Write a list of health and wellness goals you would like to achieve and put a specific date next to each one (goals without dates are just thoughts)

2. Break up the time from now to the goal date into increments (daily, weekly, monthly, quarterly)

3. Write a list of steps which, if done daily and consistently over each increment, will get you to the BIG goal

4. List bad habits or possible obstacles that might prevent you from performing the small steps daily

5. Draw from your experience in the past when you had to take consistent small steps to achieve a bigger outcome.

CHAPTER 2

MYTHS YOUR DOCTOR TOLD YOU

MYTH #1: REST UNTIL YOUR PAIN GETS BETTER

How many times have you heard your doctor or someone tell you to rest because of pain? The problem with resting until the pain gets better is that it does not address the cause of the pain. Pain is a symptom. It's your body is trying to tell you something is wrong, but that doesn't necessarily mean the painful area is the culprit. A check engine light doesn't mean there is a problem with your dashboard. Resting is like turning the car ignition off. The light goes away, but once you start the car again, it will come right back on if you haven't repaired the problem.

One client, Mary, had knee pain when she walked up and down the stairs. Our evaluation determined that her knee pain was the result of compensation from weakness in her hip muscles. Mary's knees were taking on extra pressure with every step that she walked up and down the stairs. If she stopped walking up and down the stairs, her knee pain would decrease. However, her job required walking at least 2 miles a day, and her bedroom was on the second floor of her house. Resting would not fix the cause of her knee pain, so it would always come right back. She needed to strengthen her hip muscles and keep her knees straight to reduce stress while using the stairs. If Mary were to follow her doctor's orders to rest, her leg muscles would get weaker and stiffer after several weeks; she would have been in a worse predicament then when she originally saw her doctor for the knee pain.

One of the few times that you should rest until the pain gets better is if there is structural damage such as a bone fracture. In most cases, a good PT would be able to assess the cause of your pain and create a customized solution to treat it appropriately. If it turns out that you have pain that is beyond the scope of physical therapy, we could refer you to the appropriate medical professional.

MYTH #2: DON'T LIFT OVER 25 POUNDS

When was the last time you were about to push or carry an object and stopped to weigh it? Probably never. There are only a few occasions, such as after recent surgery or heart issues, where lifting over a certain weight can cause increased problems. The human body is very resilient and strong. If trained properly, it can handle increased physical stress over time in combination with decreased risk of injury. I first met Ben 5 years after he came out of shoulder surgery. He fractured his arthritic shoulder in a fall and required a shoulder replacement. The surgeon told Ben to not lift anything greater than twenty five pounds overheard or he might damage the repair. As a grandfather, Ben was devastated that he would not be able to pick up his newborn grandson per doctor's orders. During our PT sessions, we worked on shoulder mobility and exercise technique so that he wouldn't have any issues incrementally increasing overhead motions. After 2 months of working together, Ben called to say that he picked up his grandson for the first time. He used the program I created for him and was able to strengthen his shoulders enough to lift 30 pounds overhead without any pain! His doctor was amazed.

MYTH #3: THE ONLY EXERCISE YOU NEED IS WALKING

Has your doctor ever told you that all you need to do is to walk more often? Walking is a great exercise for most people. You can do it in various settings and there is no extra equipment needed. It is primarily an endurance-based exercise. But what happens if your problems stem from a strength or balance issue? You would need a strength- or balance-related solution.

This is what happened with Paula. She was frequently falling when walking around the house. Her doctor told her to practice walking more. Her daughter was concerned because the doctor suggested Paula do more of the activity that injured her in the first place! When I first met Paula, I could tell her thigh muscles were very weak. She would take a few steps with her cane, but then her knee would buckle. The main problem with Paula was not walking. It was her leg weakness. If her leg weakness wasn't addressed, her knees would continue to buckle and falls would continue to happen no matter how much she practiced walking.

As you age, your body's endurance, strength, and balance change. Your ability to gain muscle and handle physical stress decreases. One way to counteract that is to perform weight resistance exercises. All exercises cause stress to your body. Too little stress means your body doesn't get the stimulus needed to get stronger. Too much stress puts you at risk for injury. Don't forget that walking doesn't challenge the upper body as much as the lower extremities. A customized exercise program that includes exercises for cardiovascular, strength, mobility, and balance is critical for long-term health.

MYTH #4: IT IS NORMAL AT YOUR AGE TO HAVE PAIN

Pain is a sign from your body that something is going on. However, not all pain is bad. Have you ever ramped up your activity or exercised harder than usual and found yourself sore for the next few days? This is called DOMS, delayed onset of muscle soreness. This type of soreness pain is just your muscles and body telling you that you've been working harder than usual. If you experience soreness a few days after exercising, it is actually a good thing. As the soreness goes away, the muscles get stronger and will be better equipped to handle increased stress in the future.

Other types of pain indicate negative things might be happening in your body. Dull, achy, shooting, or numb pain is not normal. If you experience any of these symptoms, please consult with your physician or PT to find the cause.

Age has nothing to do with pain. Pain does not discriminate based on age, sex, or gender. It may be true that people lead a more sedentary life as they get older, which means less exercise and decreased resistance to external stress. According to the New England Journal Of Medicine, a person who is sedentary has a greater incidence of obesity and heart disease and a higher mortality rate. A sedentary lifestyle will lead to weight gain, muscle atrophy, decreased endurance, and more stress on joints. Over time, these factors can lead to pain. Individuals who keep active and eat healthy can remain pain-free for as long as possible.

At Next Level PT, we specialize in helping individuals over 50 eliminate pain and keep it that way. Be wary next time your doctor tells you that pain is normal because of your age.

MYTH #5: YOU NEED TO STRETCH MORE

Have you ever tried stretching muscles to find that it becomes tight again after a few hours? If that's the case, stretching might not be what you need. Instead, take a look at what positions and activities your body goes through daily. If you are constantly sitting, certain muscles might be tighter versus someone who stands and walks most of the day. Imagine a contortionist and a bodybuilder on two ends of a mobility scale. The contortionist is very flexible and doesn't have a lot of bulky muscle mass; the bodybuilder is less flexible but has significantly more muscle mass. Because the contortionist has so much mobility in their body, they often lack stability in the joints; the bodybuilder has a ton of stability but lacks mobility. If you are very flexible but still have muscle tightness, it could be that your muscles are compensating by tightening up to increase stability. Muscles being tight is a symptom of an underlying issue. In order to find out why stretching is not helping your situation, reach out to my team at **nextlevelpthouston. com**. We can address your questions and concerns.

MYTH #6: SQUATTING CAN CAUSE KNEE ARTHRITIS

Arthritis means inflammation of the joint. If squatting can cause arthritis, why doesn't everybody have knee arthritis or pain as they age? There are 3 different types of arthritis: osteoarthritis, rheumatoid arthritis, and post-traumatic arthritis.

Knee osteoarthritis is the most common type and is characterized by stiffness with immobility, knee buckling, locking, swelling, and tenderness. It's what doctors mean when they say your knee is "bone-on-bone." In osteoarthritis, the cartilage between the knee wears down over time. This wearing down of the cartilage is NOT exclusive to squatting. It can occur for other reasons, such as overuse or weak supporting structures of the knee.

Rheumatoid arthritis is an autoimmune disease that causes pain throughout all the joints of the body. Symptoms include joint swelling, tenderness, pain, and stiffness. You would need a blood test and imaging to confirm this type of arthritis.

The third type of arthritis is post traumatic-arthritis. This type occurs after an injury to a joint. When a joint becomes injured, it is necessary to get the proper rehabilitation in order to strengthen the area and its surrounding structures. This will help to prevent future injuries.

The one treatment shared by all types of arthritis is exercise. Squatting is one of the best exercises you can do to combat these ailments. When performing the proper squat, it is imperative that you are aware of your knee, hip, and ankle position throughout the motion. Squatting does NOT cause knee arthritis. However, squatting improperly will put excessive stress on your knees, which can eventually lead to pain and discomfort.

If you have been diagnosed with arthritis and want to talk to a specialist about it, reach out to my team at **nextlevelpthouston.com**. We will let you know what options you have to prevent it from getting worse.

CHAPTER 3

WHAT IS THE HOLISTIC MEDICAL MODEL?

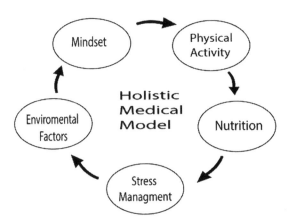

When was the last time you went to your doctor complaining of pain and left with a pain pill or recommendation for injections? That's the norm for traditional western medicine. Painkillers and injections can work wonders by reducing pain almost immediately. Unfortunately, these interventions only last for a short period of time and often have negative side effects. They create a false belief that everything is fine. Pain medications or injections temporarily block your pain symptoms, but they don't treat the real cause of it.

Let me tell you about Kevin, a 45-year-old client who has been suffering with neck pain for over 15 years. He tried pain medications, injections, and was contemplating a surgery recommended by his doctor. His x-ray and MRI showed Degenerative Disc Disease. He was desperate for alternative treatment because his friend's pain had gotten worse after neck surgery.

Kevin told me that his neck pain increased with certain movements and was worst at the end of the day. He was worried that the pain would never go away because of his degenerative disc diagnosis. What struck me most about Kevin's issue was when he said his pain increased with movement. X-rays are great at detecting bone fractures and deformities; MRIs are used to look at organs and structures of the body. None of these tests are administered when a person is moving. Finding the cause of a movement-induced pain requires a movement assessment. That's not to say x-rays and MRIs are not helpful, but imaging should not be the only test to identify an issue. My conversation with Kevin evaluated his current physical exercise, nutrition, environmental factors, stress management, and mindset about the situation. After a few months, Kevin improved all of these areas, and his chronic pain disappeared. His fears of needing surgery were no more.

After helping thousands of patients like Kevin, I created my version of the Holistic Model. The Holistic model looks at the person as a whole system and empowers people to heal themselves by treating the cause of their diseases through making lifestyle changes. The goal is to promote optimum health, which helps prevent and treat disease. We do this by focusing on five key factors: nutrition, physical activity, stress management, environmental factors, and mindset.

NUTRITION

"Our food should be our medicine and our medicine should be our food" -Hippocrates

I often get asked, "What are the best foods for me to eat?" My answer is always that it depends on your goals. Everyone's genetic makeup, body composition, and physical goals are different, so their nutritional plan should be as well. However, best practice is always to buy organic produce, which is more nutritious and has less pesticides. Here are some of the popular diets on the market today. There is no one-size-fits-all. Consult with your doctor and test to see which works best for you.

Ketogenic Diet

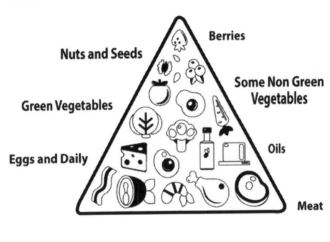

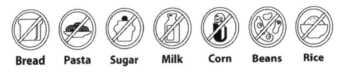

This diet consists of low-carb, high-fat consumption. When carbohydrate consumption decreases, your body reaches a stage called ketosis. During ketosis, your body burns more fat and ketones. Ketogenic diets have been shown to improve conditions such as Obesity, Diabetes, Alzheimer's, Cancer, Parkinson's, and Brain Injuries.

Foods to avoid:
- Sugary Foods
- Grains or Starches
- Beans or Legumes
- Root Vegetables
- Unhealthy Fats
- Alcohol
- Processed Foods

Foods to eat
- Meat
- Fatty Fish
- Eggs
- Cheese
- Healthy Oils
- Avocados
- Low-Carb Veggies

Mediterranean Diet

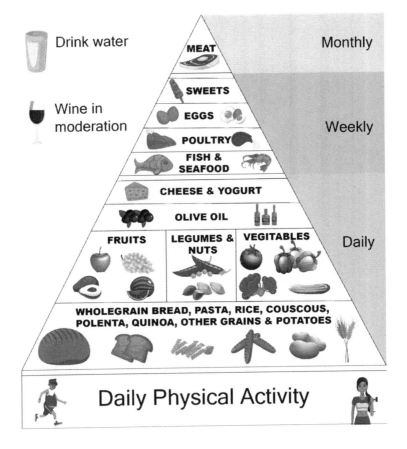

This way of eating has been shown to promote weight loss, improve cancer and diabetes prevention, and boost brain health. It emphasizes consuming cheese, fruits, nuts, vegetables, and whole grains consistently; sweets, eggs, seafood, poultry and red wine in moderation, and red meat for special occasions. Daily physical exercise and water intake are also critical for success with this program.

Gluten/Dairy/Soy Free or Elimination Diet

This diet has been gaining traction to combat food sensitivities and leaky gut syndrome. Leaky gut is a condition in which the bacteria and toxins in the digestive tract leak through the intestinal walls into the bloodstream.

The result is inflammation, bloating, fatigue, food sensitivities, or digestive issues.

Factors that can contribute to leaky gut include excessive sugar intake, long term usage of NSAIDS (non-steroidal anti-inflammatories), excessive alcohol consumption, nutrient deficiencies, stress, poor gut health, and yeast overgrowth. Be sure to get tested for food sensitivities before trying an elimination diet.

PHYSICAL ACTIVITY

Exercise has been shown to improve heart and lung function, reduce blood sugar levels, improve energy, and strengthen bones. The two main types of exercises are aerobic and muscle-strengthening.

Aerobic exercise is typically more endurance-based, which keeps the heart and lungs healthy. It is recommended to perform 150 minutes of moderate-intensity aerobic exercise per week; this includes brisk walking, dancing, or swimming. Another way to measure the intensity of the exercise is using the max heart rate formula.

Max Heart Rate = 220 - Your Age

70-80% of your max heart rate is considered moderate exercise intensity.

Muscle-strengthening exercises are great for improving your joint function and reducing risk for injury. A good strengthening program will include all major muscle groups of the body. Some popular programs include bodyweight exercises, weight training, and resistance band training. Your exercise program should be customized to fit your goals.

STRESS MANAGEMENT

Contrary to popular belief, not all stress is bad. There are two types: eustress and distress. Eustress is beneficial stress, such as exercise, receiving a job promotion, or winning money. Distress, such as divorce, injury, or financial problems, causes a negative emotional reaction. Unfortunately, we cannot escape distress indefinitely, but there are strategies to mitigate the negative side effects and increase eustress.

When your body senses distress, the hypothalamus in your brain sends signals to increase cortisol (the stress hormone). Cortisol triggers your body's fight or flight response; heart rate increases, breathing increases, and muscles are primed for action. Individuals who have prolonged exposure to distress frequently have higher cortisol levels in their system; this can lead to long-term health issues such as anxiety, depression, headaches, and insomnia.

Some strategies to reduce the effects of distress include meditation, exercise, relaxation, and social support. It is critical that you find your distress triggers in order to reduce exposure. An individual's ability to manage stress determines how well they can successfully adapt to change.

ENVIRONMENTAL FACTORS

The environment plays a huge role in your overall health. Do you get itchy eyes or a stuffy nose when there are allergens in the air? How would you feel if you were living in that environment for years? This is the story of my previous client, Jane. She was 50 years old and worked as an accountant. She complained to me of numbness in the neck and feelings of nausea that would increase whenever she was in the home for over 6 hours. Our physical therapy evaluation showed that there was nothing physically wrong with Jane, so I began to ask her questions about her home environment. She explained that she had flooding in her home 6 months ago and was still renovating the house. Jane also revealed that the numbness and nausea started a month after the flood. I suspected mold toxicity and referred her to a doctor for a test. Jane called me two weeks later saying the lab test was positive for mold. Not all health issues stem from a physical or internal trigger. Watch for patterns that increase your symptoms; this includes external triggers in your environment.

MINDSET

"If you change the way you look at things, the things you look at change."
-Wayne Dyer

What thoughts do you have about your health? When pain comes, do your thoughts stay positive or do they turn more negative? A positive mindset will push you in the right direction for recovery, but a negative mindset can hinder progression.

I met Diane after she had tried pain medications, cortisone injections, and surgery for her back pain. She was defeated mentally and only came to our PT clinic because her doctor had exhausted all other options. She thought she had tried everything else already and that PT wasn't going to work either. I challenged her on this belief, because she had never been to PT. It wasn't a bad thing that Diane had been to many different healthcare professionals without success. It meant we were now several steps closer to figuring out what actually could work. All the interventions that Diane had received previously were passive, requiring minimal commitment on her part. Physical therapy is an active approach. From the very beginning of our sessions, we set small, actionable goals. Within months, Diane achieved most of them. She went from a negative, defeatist mindset to a positive, empowered attitude as she regained control of her pain and quality of life. To this day, Diane is free from pain and living life on her terms. The first step in achieving a goal is the belief that it can be done. Once Diane believed she could take control of her situation, she thrived.

CHAPTER 4

10 SURPRISING PROBLEMS YOUR PT CAN HELP YOU WITH

PROBLEM # 1: CHRONIC PAIN

D o you know of someone who has pain that never seems to go away? They have been through pain medications, injections, or surgery, but the pain is still there. According to the Center for Disease Control, over 50 million Americans suffer from chronic pain. Common symptoms among individuals with chronic pain include weight gain, deconditioning of muscles, and increased use of medications.

Chronic pain usually starts as acute pain that never fully resolves. Over time, it develops into chronic pain. A person suffering with chronic pain may have physical dysfunctions as well as a sensitive nervous system. Every time your body senses something painful, signals get sent to the brain. The brain interprets these signals as pain, and you feel them shortly afterward. Imagine this happening everyday for months and years. When your brain is bombarded by pain signals, it forms a habit and becomes hypersensitive. It will interpret most normal sensations as unpleasant even though there is no physical damage present.

Pain starts a vicious cycle, because hypersensitive people stop moving as much. The decreased activity leads to weight gain and muscle deconditioning as well as an increased risk for heart disease and diabetes.

A physical therapist can find out if the cause of the pain is from the muscular system or from the nervous system. Once the cause is found, a customized solution can be created to resolve it. It sure beats popping endless pain pills or getting an injection that only masks the pain temporarily.

PROBLEM #2: SCAR TISSUE

Have you ever had cuts, burns, surgery, or tattoos? If so, then you have scar tissue underneath those areas. Beneath your skin is a fascial system. Fascia covers the whole body, acting as a shock absorber and helping structural integrity. When you cut a raw chicken breast, you'll see a clear, thin layer on top of the meat; that's the fascia. We all have one uniform fascia layer underneath our skin.

Your body heals through scarring. Unfortunately, scar tissue causes adhesions in the fascia which can limit range of motion, cause pain, or affect organ function. Can you imagine having scar tissue from surgery and then your surgeon tells you to get surgery again to eliminate scar tissue? The surgery that gave you scar tissue in the first place is not the solution to getting rid of it. You need a non-invasive approach such as laser, myofascial release, or MPS therapy.

My client, Jasmine, has an interesting scar tissue story. Jasmine, who is 57, had a C-section 27 years ago and her first tattoo 40 years ago. After the C-section, her low back started to get tight and she never felt the same. She had always been active when she was younger, but her low back pain became so bad over the past few years that she stopped exercising, gained weight, and couldn't even play with her grandchildren without sitting down every few minutes. She tried medications, injections, and even had her nerve blocked. None of those interventions gave her any relief. The pain medications would help for a few hours until they wore off and she had to take more. Over time, Jasmine went from taking 2 pain pills a day to 6. Her doctor recently told her she has signs of liver disease.

I explained to Jasmine how her C-section scar tissue in the front is pulling on the facial system and structures in the low back, creating tension. Our first session was for C-section scar tissue release. Jasmine had an instant decrease in pain symptoms by 50%. After all of Jasmine's scar tissue was released, she had 75% less pain for the first time in 20 years. Her pain management doctor was shocked, to say the least. The next step in her plan of care was to retrain her muscles that had atrophied over the years of being sedentary. Jasmine had developed many bad movement habits while she was trying to function with the low back pain. Now that the pain was manageable, we had to teach her how to move more efficiently to decrease excess stress on her back and other joints.

Over the next few months, Jasmine continued to get stronger, her pain pill consumption decreased, and she was able to play with her grandchildren without taking frequent breaks. One of Jasmine's triggers was tightness from post-surgical C-section scar tissue. Until it was addressed, Jasmine never stood a chance to reduce her pain symptoms. For more information on how we can help you with scar tissue issues, email us at **nextlevelpthouston@ gmail.com.**

PROBLEM #3: SCOLIOSIS

Scoliosis is a condition in which the spine is curved to the side. The 3 most common types are idiopathic, congenital, and neuromuscular. The cause of idiopathic scoliosis is unknown. Congenital scoliosis commonly results from spinal defects at birth, and neuromuscular scoliosis develops from neurological or muscular diseases such as cerebral palsy and muscular dystrophy.

The cervical, thoracic, and lumbar sections of the spine have natural curves in order to absorb and distribute the shock and load of walking, lifting overhead, jumping, or other activities. When the curves are compromised or become too prominent in one direction, it puts extra strain on the spine, muscles, and supporting structures.

The body works by compensation. Think of the last time you hurt one arm. How did you get by? You probably used the opposite arm until the injured arm stopped hurting. The same concept applies to the muscles that keep your spine stable throughout different movements. If your spine is curved more toward the left, the muscles on your left have to work harder to prevent the spine from going that way too much. This might help for a little while, but then the muscles start to fatigue. That is when problems such as back pain, stiffness, and achiness arise. Don't forget that the spine is all connected, even though there are 3 different sections. What happens to one section of the spine will affect the other sections as well.

At Next Level PT, we categorize clients with scoliosis as having a structural or functional scoliosis. Client with structural scoliosis have a curvature so prominent that they require or have already had scoliosis surgery. Clients with functional scoliosis have developed a relatively minor curvature as a result of poor postural habits or repetitive movements. Regardless of whether you have a functional or structural scoliosis, we always assess how your body is moving, analyze any compensation, and determine whether it is efficient. Then we can strengthen the supporting structures of the spine in order to prevent the scoliosis from increasing over time.

One of my clients, Debbie, had a remarkable scoliosis journey. Debbie developed scoliosis in her teenage years and required Harrington rods to stop her curvature from progressing. These rods straighten the curve of the spine at the expense of spine flexibility. Her doctor told her that she had to keep her weight under 130lbs and that she'd never be able to walk for longer than a mile without pain. What a scary thought to be told by your doctor that you'll have pain for the rest of your life at such a young age!

I first met Debbie when she was 60 years old and the owner of a successful wedding photography business. She complained of an achy, stiff back pain when moving her heavy camera equipment. The daily pain medications weren't working anymore, and she wanted a natural solution for her problems. Her orthopedic surgeon told her she might need surgery again to realign the rods. In our discovery session, we were able to see that her body was compensating poorly because of uneven weight distribution and that she had faulty movement patterns when moving heavy objects. After several weeks of working with Debbie, her pain went from a constant 8 out of 10 to a 0 by following our customized postural and strengthening program. At the next appointment, her surgeon told that she no longer required surgery.

Today, eight months after her first appointment, Debbie is still free of back pain. She is able to walk 2 miles a day with her husband and dogs without having to sit down every few minutes. She feels "in control of her life" and no longer has to resort to pain medications just to get through the day.

PROBLEM #4: MIGRAINES/HEADACHES

When was the last time you had a migraine at the end of the day or when performing a specific task? Did your doctor prescribe a painkiller or order a scan to rule out any brain abnormalities? Painkillers can temporarily relieve headaches, but if the cause is from a muscular- or nerve-related issue, medications alone won't work. Most of the people that come to Next Level PT for chronic migraines have already tried medications, different diets, and staying hydrated without long-term results. It's important to track when the migraine is present and what activities led up to it. Is it during a particular time of day or after a period of time in a certain body position? The more information we have about your migraine triggers, the better we are able to create your customized solution.

Robert came to Next Level PT having suffered with chronic headaches for 15 years. He worked for a doctor's office as a medical assistant, so he would spend 8 hours a day entering patient data on the computer. His boss, the doctor, prescribed him pain medications and told him to drink more water. Robert tried this strategy for a few years until that stopped helping. He started to get tingling and numbness shoot down his arms along with neck pain after a long day at work. He noticed the pattern of symptoms getting worse toward the end of the day.

I told Robert to have his colleague take a picture of him at his workstation. The picture showed that Robert's laptop screen was too low, so that he was looking down a majority of the time. This position causes excessive stress on the neck bones and muscles. He moved his screen up to eye level, and his headache symptoms dropped 25% from that change alone!

Robert also had very stiff neck muscles from the years from sitting in the same position every day. We worked on his sitting posture and loosened up his neck muscles to regain normal, pain-free movement. After 4 months of working on stretching, strengthening, and postural training, Robert's 15 years of migraines are no more. Pain medications and drinking more water would have never solved his chronic migraine issue. No x-ray, MRI, or CT scan would show that posture and tight, weak muscles were the major cause. It took a physical therapist who listened, asked the right questions, and figured out what Robert was doing outside the clinic that triggered the issues.

PROBLEM #5: BALANCE

Have you fallen in the last year? Do you lose your balance frequently? We ask these questions to all our clients with muscular, inner ear, or neurological dysfunctions. Balance is a skill just like walking or jumping. As babies, we gain the skill of balance through repetitive practice of standing, falling, walking, falling, etc. until we can move around without issues.

A fall or loss of balance can disrupt your confidence in being mobile and independent. Some common things we hear from clients are:

- My balance is bad because of my age
- I can't walk without a walker or cane
- I fall a lot, but I'm not sure what to do about it

Age and decline of balance are not correlated. Balance is a skill. If not worked on, it will get worse over time. Imagine a basketball player shooting 500 jump shots a day, taking a year off of basketball, and then trying to shoot 500 shots again. Chances are they won't make as many when they come back.

Most of the clients we see with balance dysfunctions have a problem with muscle weakness. If your leg muscles are weak or stiff, then you're going to have difficulty walking without losing your balance. A cane or walker might help in the short term, but strengthening and stretching exercises are necessary to treat the cause. People who have a history of falls tend to stop moving as much due to fear of falling again. This is actually the worst thing to do. When you stop moving because of fear, the muscles in the body become even stiffer and weaker. You might also gain more weight due to inactivity. Do you see how this can become a continuous cycle?

The inner ear is another common source for increased fall risk. The inner ear has three components, called the vestibule, cochlea, and semicircular canals. There are crystals, fluid, and sensors in the inner ear that move with your body or head position, giving your brain the information necessary to maintain balance.

A common inner ear condition called BPPV (benign paroxysmal positional vertigo) causes dizziness when there is a disruption between the crystals, fluid, and sensors. Just imagine the sensors in your ear telling your brain that you're standing upright but your eyes are telling it that you are lying down. The brain can't decide between these two conflicting messages, so vertigo and dizziness occur. One quick way to test for BPPV is to see if your symptoms go away with your eyes closed. When you close your eyes, the brain is only receiving information from the inner ear regarding head position, so there will no longer be a conflict and vertigo symptoms will go away until you open the eyes again.

Neurological problems such as multiple sclerosis, parkinson disease, stroke, and diabetes can cause balance deficits as well. These diagnoses can affect sensation in the feet and the brain-to-muscle connection. When brain-to-muscle communication is affected, the muscles do not work with the necessary quickness or strength.

My client, Tom, sustained a mild stroke at the age of 48 due to a blood clot in his brain. He was an avid runner, but afterward he had trouble just walking because the left side of his body was so weak. When he walked, his left foot wouldn't clear the floor. With each step, you could hear the foot dragging. This increased his fall risk exponentially. Luckily for Tom, he came to Next Level PT, where we were able to teach him and his spouse strategies on how to improve strength on the left side of the body as well as the brain-to-muscle connection. One year later, Tom is back to walking again without any issues.

PROBLEM #6: OSTEOARTHRITIS

Have you ever been to your doctor with pain and told that you have arthritis or that the joint is "bone-on-bone"? One of the most common things we hear from our new clients is, "My doctor told me surgery is the only option because my joint is bone-on-bone." It may be true that an x-ray or MRI shows damage to the cartilage, but there's no guarantee that surgery will fix the problem. Osteoarthritis is another word for inflammation of the joint. Inflammation is a symptom. The question is why the inflammation is there in the first place. There can be several factors that cause joint inflammation, including weak muscles, how the joint is used, and nutrition.

One client we helped with knee arthritis was Mike. He was 44 years old and loved to play basketball and golf. He'd play on the weekends with his friends as a way to de-stress from the work week. Unfortunately, Mike also had knee pain every time he jumped or swung his golf club. At the doctor, he was given an x-ray and told he had knee arthritis. The doctor prescribed pain medications and recommended surgery if the knee was still bothering him in 6 months. Mike was devastated at the thought of potentially needing knee surgery. His grandmother had knee surgery at 76 years old and was never able to walk the same again.

During our PT evaluation, Mike had no pain with walking or squatting; it was only present with landing from a jump or twisting the knee during a swing. When we focused on these two specific activities, we found the cause of the pain. Every time Mike would jump and land, his knees would shift inwards, knocking into each other. He was also putting too much stress on the lead knee when swinging a club. The combination of these faulty movement patterns over time caused the knee to take on extra stress. After 2 months of correcting Mike's landing and swinging technique, he is pain free. He no longer needs knee surgery because we treated the real cause of his knee pain rather than just the symptoms of inflammation.

We treat people like Mike every day, but we also see clients who are in worse scenarios after their doctors label them as having "bone-on-bone" arthritis. These people have pain with almost all motions, so they stop moving as much to prevent the pain from increasing. Unfortunately, this strategy can lead to weight gain, increased joint stiffness, and muscle atrophy. This means more pain and difficulty with movement!

Susan called my office because she kept falling at home. Her doctor said she had "low back bone-on-bone arthritis." Susan was 63 years old and newly retired from a desk job in corporate America. She used to walk her dog everyday with her husband as a form of exercise. Over the past 2 years, however, her low back pain worsened so much that she was forced to give up her daily walks. She started to gain weight, and it was harder to get around the house.

My first few sessions with Susan included education on exercise and ways to offset pressure on her low back. She was resistant to move because of pain, yet she reported feeling looser after moving. It was a question of short-term gain for long-term pain or short-term pain for long-term gain. Susan chose the latter. She wanted to walk the dogs with her husband again. She realized that learning how to move again might be painful at first but that it would get better if she stuck with it. I encouraged Susan's husband to join our sessions as her accountability partner.

If you are suffering from osteoarthritis and you've been told that surgery is the only option, please seek a more conservative approach such as physical therapy. A good PT clinic can help you avoid unnecessary surgery!

PROBLEM #7: TMJ IMPAIRMENTS

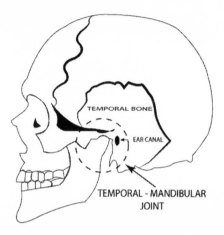

The TMJ, or temporomandibular joint, is the hinge that connects the jawbone to the skull. Clients with TMJ issues present with locking of the jaw, pain while chewing, or facial pain.

One of my clients, Jill, had TMJ problems for over 5 years. She had neck pain and difficulty chewing. Her oral surgeon started her on a mouth guard, pain medications, and then injections. During our examination, I found clicking on the jaw every time she opened and closed her mouth. No wonder she had pain. Her TMJ was moving too much, pulling at the jaw and neck muscles. Medications and injections were just treating the inflammation and pain, not the unstable TMJ. After several sessions of massage to calm down the TMJ muscles, I taught Jill jaw strengthening exercises. Her TMJ stopped clicking, and the surrounding muscles were no longer getting pulled. Jill also had a slouched sitting posture, which affected the neck and jaw muscles. We worked on sitting and standing posture with methods to decompress the neck muscles. This allowed the jaw to be in the proper position every time Jill chewed. After 2 months, the jaw and neck pain subsided, so she no longer needs her mouth guard throughout the day.

If you have jaw pain like Jill, contact our PT clinic at **nextlevelpthouston. com**. We can help you find and treat the cause naturally without medications or injections.

PROBLEM #8: CONCUSSION

Have you ever sustained trauma to your head where you suffered temporary loss of consciousness, confusion, ringing in the ears, or dizziness? If so, you might have post-concussion symptoms. A concussion is a brain injury that occurs when there is a blow to the head. Treatments for concussion include vision therapy, balance therapy, physical therapy, and cognitive behavioral therapy. The different types of therapy are directly correlated with the dysfunctions of the post-concussion client. At Next Level PT, we specialize in treating concussion using microcurrent point stimulation to heal the brain. Our concussion recovery therapy protocol helps improve circulation to the brain, which has been shown to decrease post-concussion symptoms and promote healing.

Sally was 54 years old when she sustained a stroke. The left side of her body became weak, so she went to a hospital physical therapy office for balance and gait training. Three months later, Sally fell when trying to get out of her car and sustained a concussion. She fell into a coma for months. Her doctor recommended pulling the plug, but the family kept fighting, and Sally woke up three weeks later. She had constant dizziness, headaches, neck pain, and an extreme fear of falling. Sally went to a local physical therapy office, where she was treated for her post-concussion symptoms, but after four months of treatment, her symptoms remained the same. She was still unable to stand unassisted because of the dizziness, and her neck pain caused her to look down at the floor when attempting to walk.

Sally was referred to Next Level PT by a friend who we helped recover from concussion symptoms. Looking at Sally's therapy history, we realized there was very little done for her brain. Most of the treatment she received was managing the symptoms. After six sessions of our comprehensive concussion recovery protocol, Sally's dizziness and headaches disappeared. She still had neck pain and a fear of falling, however, so the next phase of treatment was getting rid of the neck issues by re-learning postures in sitting, standing, and walking. Once the pain was gone, it was just a matter of time until Sally regained the strength and confidence to walk again.

Today, Sally is walking without any assistive device and spends her weekends playing with the grandchildren. Her story shows how important it is after a concussion to heal the brain before working on the symptoms.

If you or a loved one is suffering from concussion symptoms and would like to know your options, reach out to my team at **nextlevelpthouston. com**. We will put you in touch with our concussion specialist.

PROBLEM #9: ATHLETIC PERFORMANCE

Do you play sports or exercise? If yes, have you ever used a coach to improve your performance? A good PT can help with injury prevention and also find and fix movement impairments that limit your athletic performance.

One of my clients, Paul, is an avid golfer. Paul is 58 years old, works a desk job, and plays golf three times a week. For the past few years, Paul's golf score has been stagnant, and he's noticed the mid and low back hurting after each session. His golf coach referred Paul to my clinic when the pain caused his swing not to be fluid. During our evaluation, I found that Paul had limited mobility in the mid and low back, but he was forcing rotation (which he lacked) every time he swung the club. That's why his back was tight and painful after each golf session. We created a program to increase mobility in his back and correct his swing. He gained awareness of how different body positions throughout the day can add extra stress to the back. Within 2 months, Paul's score improved 10 strokes and his back stopped hurting. If you're frustrated with your athletic performance and want to improve, start with your coach to find the restrictions and then work with a physical therapist to resolve them.

PROBLEM #10: QUALITY OF LIFE

"It is not the years in your life that count, it is the life in your years."

According to a study by Canadian Medical Association Journal, physical exercise has been shown to cut risk of early death by 50%. As people age, the risk of injuries and falls increases. However, contrary to popular belief, not all exercises are created equal.

When was the last time you tried achieving a goal without guidance or directions? You probably had a difficult time, but the majority of people who call our clinic for help do just that. They exercise without proper guidance. Maybe they watch a Youtube video exercise and injure themselves. Maybe they were told to walk more, the most common exercise doctors prescribe. Unfortunately, for many people over 50, walking is simply not enough to keep their body resilient against future injures.

You perform various tasks, such as carrying, lifting, squatting, and jumping every day. Why are you not training in the same manner? Proper exercise programming from a physical therapist can help your body build muscle to cushion external forces and improve performance during daily activities.

Susan was 68 years old and an avid walker who walked 2 miles a day when she broke her hip during a fall in her house. Her doctor recommended walking more as a solution. A few months later, Susan was still limping and unable to walk a mile. Frustrated with the doctor's orders, she found Next Level PT. We assessed her movement and fall risk. Susan's biggest weakness was standing up from a seated position. Once she was standing, she had an easier time getting around.

The reason why walking didn't work is that it was addressing a problem she didn't have. We worked with Susan to improve her squat movement, balance, and strength in the lower extremities. As of today, Susan is walking 2 miles a day without any pain or limp. When we asked Susan what kept her so consistent with her PT visits, she said, "My mother fell in her 60s and her doctor told her to walk more, but she never recovered fully, so I knew that I needed more."

Susan's story is one of hundreds that we hear in the clinic. A fall risk problem requires a fall risk program. With the proper customized solution, Susan was able to perform the task that gives her joy and decrease her chance for future falls.

CHAPTER 5

NECK PAIN

Neck pain is one of the most common issues we help solve in our clinic. The causes can range from poor postural habits such as sitting hunched over staring at your phone to whiplash from a car accident to muscular strains from exercise. Structural deficits such as arthritis or cervical stenosis are also a possibility. In most cases, neck pain doesn't occur overnight unless it is from a whiplash, strain from muscle overexertion, or direct trauma to the neck. Instead, small tensions build up over time into a serious problem.

Have you ever noticed increased stiffness in your neck after a long day at work or sitting for prolonged periods of time? Are you aware of your posture or neck position? How often are you stretching and relaxing the neck muscles throughout the day?

The next time you are at work or in a public place, take a look at the sitting and standing neck posture of people around you. You will notice a dramatic difference between each individual. While I don't believe there is a "perfect posture" because everybody's physique is different, there are ways to improve posture to decrease extra stress on the neck and spine muscles.

HOW YOUR PHONE IS CONTRIBUTING TO YOUR NECK PAIN

As technology improves and our phones get "smarter," with more applications to make life more convenient, our usage skyrockets. Over the past 20 years, the incidence of non-traumatic-related neck pain is also increasing in younger adults. Many of our clients with neck pain have previously worked a desk job, hunched over for prolonged periods, or are constantly on their phone, developing a forward head posture.

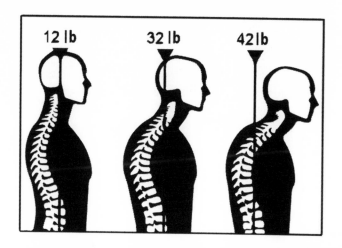

The average head weighs around 12 pounds. Think of your spine as bricks of different thickness stacked on top of each other. The more uniform the bricks are stacked, the stronger the foundation. The thinner bones are under the skull. As you move closer to the lower back, the bones are thicker because they need to support all the weight above it. When you develop forward head posture, the bones in the neck area are shifted forward, causing the head's center of mass to shift in the same direction, which in turn causes the neck and upper back muscles to be compressed and stretched. As time passes, the weight of the head puts extra stress on the neck bones.

Doing this once or twice a day for short periods of time most likely won't cause any major issues. Most of the people who have forward head posture have developed a habit of being in that position for months and years without realizing it! They might start feeling increased achy or dull pain in the neck after a long day at work that never goes away. This continues until they are forced to go to the doctor's office for neck pain that has become so unbearable it begins to affect their sleep or daily function. Sounds like a scary thought, but this is exactly what happened to our client, Lisa.

LISA'S NECK PAIN

When I first got an email from Lisa, she told me that she has been dealing with neck pain for over 20 years. She had finally contacted me because the pain was "taking over her life." Lisa was 61 years old, a dentist hygienist by trade, and the mom of 2 dogs. She explained her typical work day as cleaning teeth for 8 hours followed by doing notes for 2 hours on her laptop. During her downtime, she liked to walk her dogs and do yoga. Now she could only work 4 hours and was forced to hire a dog walker and give up yoga.

Lisa had started to experience "dull and achy neck pain" while in dental hygienist school. She would regularly see a massage therapist to alleviate her neck tension. After dental hygienist school, she continued to have neck pain, which got worse when she started working longer hours. Over the years, her doctor gave her muscle relaxants, creams, and injections for the pain. Her recent x-ray showed degeneration of the bones, which is normal for someone in their 60s. Lisa went to a chiropractor for neck adjustments, but she only felt better for a few hours before the pain came back. She also tried a massage therapist and an acupuncturist with no long-term relief. Her doctor decided to increase her pain medication dosage and told her to come back in four weeks if her symptoms didn't change.

Lisa felt stuck. She had listened to her primary doctor all these years, took the medications on time, went for injections, and applied the creams faithfully. Yet she found no significant pain relief. All she wanted to do was work effectively and walk her dogs without any limitations. This is why pain medications usually do more harm than good. They mask the pain and give the client false hope that everything is fine, at least until they wear off. That's when the real trouble sets in. When you feel less pain, you most likely will do more of the things that the pain was limiting you from, not realizing the increased activity will cause more stress to the already irritated areas. Not to mention all the negative side effects and stress to your internal organs with each pain medication you ingest.

Unsurprisingly, Lisa's neck pain didn't get any better with the increased pain medication dosage. After four weeks, Lisa's physician wanted to switch the pain medication to another type (which Lisa knew was not the solution) and refer her to a spine surgeon for further options.

When Lisa saw the surgeon, he took an X-ray and MRI to see if surgery was needed. Results showed that her neck problems were not serious enough to need surgery, so she was referred to physical therapy in the same building for three times a week for five weeks. When asked about her treatments, Lisa told me, "The therapist would ask me questions for 15 minutes about my neck pain for that day, and then give me a sheet of neck exercises to do in the gym area by myself. He would tell me to reach out to his assistants after I finished. At the end of the session, the assistant would put a heat pack on my neck followed by a ten minute massage. This happened every session."

Unfortunately, this is a common scenario we hear from clients who've been to previous physical therapy. Many in-network PT clinics operate by seeing as many patients as possible at the expense of spending more time with each client to give them a customized program tailored to their issues. After five weeks of cookie cutter PT, the surgeon took another MRI and recommended Lisa get surgery. Fortunately, this is where Lisa decided enough was enough. She had been listening to her doctors and going along with their plans for years, but her situation was still the same if not worse. She decided to do her own research to find someone who would listen to her needs and give her an option that didn't involve more medications or surgery.

Lisa saw my clinic through a local event. She was interested in the neck pain guide we offered but didn't request it because she wasn't sure physical therapy could help her. Given her previous experience, it's no wonder that she was skeptical.

After finding our clinic online, Lisa read the reviews and checked out the video testimonials from our previous clients. One of the videos was of a woman suffering from neck pain for years, just as Lisa had. She emailed us, and we set her up for a discovery session to address her questions and concerns free of charge! She had finally found a clinic that would help her regain control over her life.

The Real Cause Of Lisa's Neck Pain

After listening to Lisa's story, I explained how she had most likely developed forward head posture from her dental hygienist school days and long study sessions. When you are hunched over, studying for long periods of time with your head down and shoulders rounded, the neck muscles get compressed and stressed. Lisa was never made aware of this and never worked with a physical therapist to correct her posture, so this became her normal postural habit. She would be in the forward head posture whenever she commuted, sat on the couch at home, or worked at her office. It's not a surprise that her neck muscles were stressed and angry at her after all these years.

The doctor's solution of muscle relaxants and injections failed because it only masked the pain symptoms instead of treating the real cause. Medications or injections won't teach Lisa how to get out of the forward head position or stretch her muscles to soothe them. This is exactly what Lisa needed to treat the cause and reverse 20 years of stress and pressure on her neck.

The first step in helping Lisa was releasing her tight neck muscles to decrease the pain. Every time Lisa turned her head, the neck pain would increase. She was hesitant to move her neck because of this. When she drove, her neck muscles would tighten in anticipation of the pain kicking in. Once Lisa's muscle tension was eliminated, the next step was to teach her proper postural mechanics.

The first step in solving any problem is awareness. Lisa was never aware she was in the forward head posture all these years, so I had to retrain her brain to recognize bad postural habits. As you can imagine, changing a 20-year habit takes longer than one to two sessions. It took Lisa two months to become an expert on feeling the difference between forward head posture and her optimal posture position, which varies with every client. We also created a customized program for Lisa to strengthen her neck muscles to speed up the recovery process. Once Lisa had no more pain and her neck muscles had optimal strength, the next step was the tune up phase.

In this phase, we created a game plan to prevent any future neck pain. Shortly after our PT sessions, Lisa went back to the surgeon with no neck pain and an improved awareness of optimal sitting and standing posture. She no longer needed surgery and was able to resume yoga and walking her dogs without limitations.

HOW TO TEST AND FIX FORWARD HEAD POSTURE

The Test:

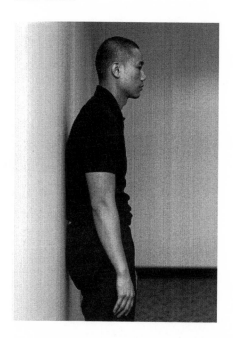 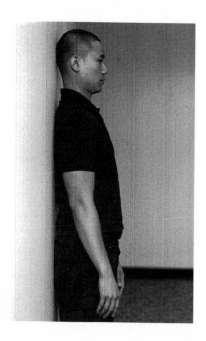

All you need to test your own head posture is a wall. Stand with your heels, butt, and shoulder blades touching the wall. There should be a slight arch in the low back. Now try to touch the wall with the back of your head without tilting your head up or increasing the low back arch. If you can't do this, you most likely have muscle imbalances of the neck and forward head posture.

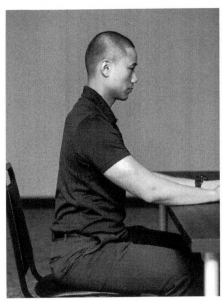 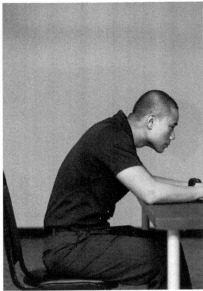

The Fix:

Take a look at the pictures above. Can you tell which one is a forward head position? There are 2 main things to note. The first is the neck jutting out and tilted upwards like a turtle sticking its head up out of its shell. The second is the excessive curvature (flexion) of the thoracic spine. In order to fix forward head posture, you need to loosen the tight neck muscles, sit up tall, bring both shoulders back, keep the chin tucked in, and improve extension of the mid back.

Here are some common stretches we teach our clients with chronic neck pain:

SCM (Sternocleidomastoid) Stretch

To perform a SCM stretch on the right side of the neck, sit up tall and pull the right side of the collarbone down toward the hip. Turn your head to the left 4 inches, and then tilt your head back. You should feel the stretch from behind the right ear towards the right collarbone. Hold this position for 30-60 seconds and repeat 3x a day. To stretch the left SCM, pull the left side of the collarbone down toward the hip. Turn your head to the right 4 inches, and then tilt your head back.

Levator Scapulae Stretch

To perform the left levator scapulae stretch, sit up tall and prop your straight left arm up on a wall. Turn your head 4 inches to the right, and with your right hand, pull the back of your head toward the outside of your right knee. Hold this position for 30-60 seconds and repeat 3x a day. To stretch the right levator scapulae, prop your straight right arm up on a wall, turn your head 4 inches to the left, and use your left hand to pull the back of your head toward the outside of your left knee.

Mid Back Extension Stretch

In a chair with a backrest, put a rolled up towel horizontally in the mid back area between the shoulder blades. Put both hands behind the ears, and then lean up, over, and backwards. The analogy I often use is imagine you're an Olympic high jumper and the towel is the stick that you have to jump over backwards. You don't want to bend into the stick; you want to jump up and over the stick in order to avoid being disqualified. You should feel the stretch in your back muscles as well as your chest and stomach muscles. Hold this position for up to 1 minute at a time.

Suboccipital Muscle Release

These are the muscles right under the back ridge of your skull that connect to the neck. Most people with forward head posture hold a lot of tension in this area and complain of achiness and soreness. You can put a lacrosse ball under the ridge of the skull and lie flat on your back. The pressure of the lacrosse ball on the suboccipital muscles can increase soreness in the neck temporarily. If that is the case, you have hit a muscle knot. Apply direct pressure into the sore spot with the ball and move your neck side to side massage out the suboccipital muscle to decrease tension. Perform on both sides of the neck for 2 minutes each.

Chin Tuck

Sit in a comfortable chair where your pelvis doesn't sink in. Imagine there is a tennis ball between the bottom of your chin and the top of your collar bone. Squeeze this imaginary ball. If done properly, you should feel a tightening of the muscles under the chin and also a stretch in the neck muscles on the back of your head. Another way to perform the chin tuck is to imagine there is a pin that goes from the outside of one ear to the outside of the other ear. Your chin is rotating down on this pin. The correct motion is the chin sliding towards the back of your neck then rotating down toward the collarbone. Some of my clients describe it as creating a "double chin." One of the biggest mistakes I see people do when learning the chin tuck is excessive cervical retraction. This will cause the neck bones to slide too much on top of each other, therefore, increasing shearing forces and cause irritation to the bones.

Here are some of the common neck diagnoses people with neck pain have:

Bulging discs and Herniation

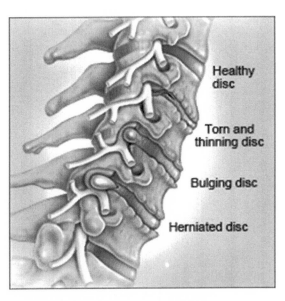

Healthy disc

Torn and thinning disc

Bulging disc

Herniated disc

In the picture above, you can see the difference between healthy, bulging, and herniated discs of the neck bones (cervical). The main function of the intervertebral discs is to absorb shock for the spine. Discs can bulge from disc degeneration over time, injury, or poor postural habits. A bulging disc is a precursor to a herniated disc if left untreated. Symptoms of herniated disc in the neck include neck pain and tingling or numbness from the shoulders down toward the fingers.

Cervical Stenosis

Cervical Stenosis occurs when there is narrowing of the space between the vertebral bones. It can be caused by disc bulges, spine degeneration, or bone spurs. People with neck stenosis often feel pain when looking up toward the sky and numbness or tingling shooting down the shoulders and fingers. Nerve symptoms for stenosis and herniated discs overlap, so it is critical to find a physical therapist that specializes in spinal dysfunctions to differentiate the cause.

Whiplash

Whiplash occurs when the neck muscles are strained from a rapid, uncontrolled movement. This can happen due to a motor vehicle accident, impact from sports, or a fall. Common symptoms include neck pain, headaches, pain or numbness in hands, and dizziness. If you have suffered an impact to the head or neck, it is also important to be assessed for concussion symptoms. X-rays and MRIs may not show the effects of whiplash. A proper whiplash assessment should include neck movement and strength test. In most cases, pain medications, injections, or surgery aren't required for treatment.

SEVEN SIMPLE TIPS TO STOP NECK PAIN FROM DISTURBING SLEEP AND CAUSING SEVERE HEADACHES

Tip #1: Get a Custom Pillow

Did you know that you spend one third of your life sleeping? You wouldn't wear a one-size-fits-all shirt, so why would you use a one-size-fits-all pillow? You want to purchase a pillow that is measured to your neck circumference, shoulder width, and neck height. Everything we provide at Next Level PT is customized, so contact us at **www.nextlevelpthouston.com** to get measured for your custom pillow for a better night sleep.

Tip# 2: Be Aware Of Your Sitting Posture

When sitting, don't slouch. This position can put unnecessary stress on your spine all the way up to your neck. Sit on your "sit bones," which are the bony prominences on your buttock.

An appropriate sitting position will allow your spine to be better equipped to withstand external forces and your joints to move more freely. If you are working on a computer, make sure you are able to touch the screen when sticking your hand in front of you. When looking straight ahead, your eyes should be looking at the middle of the screen.

Tip# 3: Don't Use Your Electronic Devices In Bed

Poor postural habits form when you constantly look down at devices, which can accumulate into excess muscle tension and neck pain.

Many people browse and play on their devices in bed before falling asleep. Propping pillows underneath the head to get a better look at your device can do more harm than you think. Your neck is not structured to be held in an upward position for prolonged periods of time. Holding these awkward neck postures can lead to muscle imbalances, trigger points, structural changes, and injuries.

Tip# 4: Use A Headset For Phone Calls

Do you bend your head to the side to hold a phone between your shoulder and ears? If so, you are asking for trouble.

You want to keep your neck and shoulder posture as symmetrical as possible. Headsets will allow you to keep your head upright while decreasing pressure, strain, and discomfort on your neck muscles.

Tip# 5: Use Ice Or Heat

Ice or heat can help to decrease inflammation and provide pain relief. If your neck pain is tender, achy, sore or pulsating, ice or heat will reduce these inflammatory responses within the muscles. Use gel or hot and cold packs for 10-15 minutes every hour as needed.

Tip #6: Stretch Daily

If you sit for prolonged periods, your neck can become stiff or tight. It is recommended to stretch your neck every hour to relieve tension and keep your muscles mobile. Stretches should be held for 30 seconds to 1 minute.

Tip #7: Alternate Carrying Your Purse or Bag Between Shoulders

If you're consistently carrying heavy objects on one shoulder, it can lead to muscle imbalances. You want to use a backpack when possible to distribute equal weight throughout the body. When more muscles work together, the chance of one muscle overworking is significantly decreased.

Tight upper back muscles can refer pain to your neck. Keeping your posture symmetrical will prevent overuse and repetitive injuries from occurring.

If you are suffering with neck pain and would like some guidance or need your questions and concerns answered, reach out to my team at **nextlevelpthouston.com**. Our neck pain specialist would love to speak with you.

CHAPTER 6

SHOULDER PAIN

Shoulder pain is one of the main reasons our clients are forced to modify exercise or daily tasks. We use our shoulders for many movements, from pull ups and pushups to carrying a grocery bag to reaching upward to put a dish in the cupboard. How many tasks have you done today that required shoulder movement?

The shoulder is the most flexible joint in the body, so it requires more stability compared to other joints. Every major joint in the body has two types of muscles: stabilization muscles and power muscles. The responsibility of the shoulder stabilization muscles is to keep the shoulder joint in the socket throughout motion. There are four of them, and together they are called the rotator cuff muscles. The power muscles of the shoulder are the deltoid muscles, which are primarily used during heavier everyday activities such as lifting or pulling.

What makes the shoulder joint complex is there are several moving parts. In order for the shoulder to have normal, unrestricted movement, you need the spine, shoulder joint, and shoulder blade muscles to work together as a team. I always describe the shoulder joint as a pulley system that sits between the shoulder blade (scapula) and the forearm. Every time you hold your cell phone next to your ear, the muscles in the shoulder blade, shoulder joint, and forearm work together to bring your hand up toward your face. If one of these muscles or joints is compromised, other muscles will have to compensate in order to perform the task.

Many of our clients come in with complaints of shoulder achiness, pain, or stiffness. One of the examinations we do at Next Level PT is to assess each part of the "shoulder pulley system" to make sure each component has adequate stability and mobility. More often than not there is a fault in one part of the system, which causes the other parts to compensate and take on more stress. In this case, an x-ray or an MRI might show arthritis, a rotator cuff tear, or bone spurs, but there are many things you can do naturally, without surgery, to slow this process and keep your shoulder functioning well into your elderly years.

Our recent client, May, learned this the hard way. May is 49 years old and has been an athlete all her life. She's a librarian who lifts weights three to four times a week and runs on the weekends. One day she felt a pull in her shoulder while carrying books. Next thing she knew, she had sharp pain every time she tried to lift the arm overhead. She'd always had sore and achy shoulders after exercises, but this time it felt different.

May went for a massage a few days later to relax the sore shoulder area, but the muscle sensitivity increased. A friend recommended a chiropractor for spine and shoulder adjustments, but after four sessions, she still had sharp pain with overhead motions. Her primary doctor gave her muscle relaxants, but those caused her to become drowsy during work. All this time, she continued to work out by modifying the exercises and avoiding the painful motions.

Three months passed, and the shoulder pain kept getting worse. Her shoulder function and range of motion kept declining until she was forced to stop exercising. That was her turning point. She researched shoulder solutions and was intrigued how Next Level PT assessed the whole shoulder system before creating a customized plan to fix it. At our discovery session, we discovered how every time May carried books, she would round and shrug her shoulders. This bad habit caused uneven pull on her shoulder and neck muscles, which led to an imbalance in her shoulder pulley system.

We also discovered some underutilized shoulder blade muscles. May had a combination of movement and strength dysfunction. This was most likely due to years of poor lifting techniques. She was suffering from a condition called anterior shoulder impingement syndrome. One of the ways this occurs is that the arm bone (humerus) jams into the front of the shoulder blade bone (acromion) during arm movement. As the bones jam into each other, the rotator muscles in between get pinched, causing sharp pain.

If the muscles get pinched once or twice, there is no permanent damage, but if they are repeatedly pinched for a prolonged period of time, there can be muscle tears. Fortunately for May, she came to us before any tears were present. The first phase of treatment was to educate her on a safe way to carry and lift books overhead onto a bookshelf. Next, we strengthened her shoulder stabilization muscles so that her body could tolerate days in which she has to carry and lift heavier books. After 3 weeks, her shoulder pain was gone and she was back to lifting weights and carrying books at work.

When May graduated from our physical therapy transformation phase to the tune-up phase, she reflected on all the treatments she had prior to coming to Next Level PT. She realized that everyone else she saw was addressing only one part of her shoulder system. That's why she was only getting temporary relief. We addressed the whole system and rebalanced it so the pain was gone for good.

If you have been diagnosed with anterior shoulder impingement like May, here are several exercises that can help reduce stress on the shoulder joint:

Chest Stretch over Foam Roller

Lie face up with your spine along the length of the foam roller. Bend both knees to take stress off the low back area. Keep both arms straight with palms facing the sky and then let it relax into the floor. If done correctly, you should feel a stretch in the chest and front of the shoulder. Hold this position for up to 1 minute.

W Pulls with Theraband

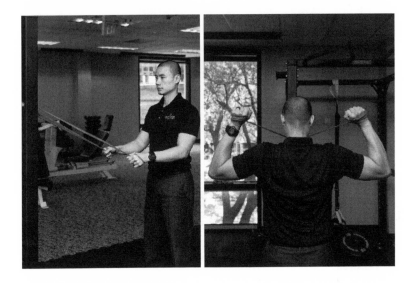

Stand up tall. Tie a band directly at your shoulder level. Grab the band with both palms facing the floor with elbows bent and pull it toward your face. As you pull the band, turn both forearms and palms back. The ending position of the palms should be facing forward in the same direction as your face, with your arms and neck forming a W shape. You should feel the muscles tighten behind the shoulder as well as the shoulder blades.

Serratus Punches

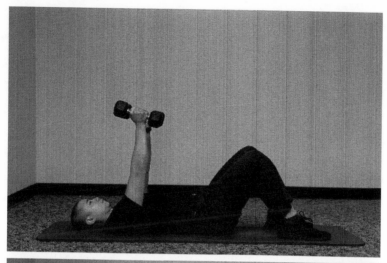

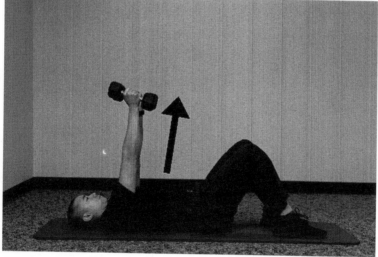

Lie on your back with both of your arms straight, pointing toward the ceiling, and both knees bent. Hold a weight in each hand. Move both arms up toward the ceiling, keeping your elbows straight out, and try to lift your shoulder blades off the floor. As you perform this exercise, try envisioning your shoulder blades spreading away from the mid back.

COMMON SHOULDER DIAGNOSES

At Next Level PT, we treat all kinds of shoulder issues. Here are some of the most common problems we work with:

Rotator Cuff Tear

The shoulder joint lacks stability because of all the mobility that it has, meaning the four rotator cuff muscles have to work hard to keep the shoulder in its socket every time you use your arm for a task. Like every muscle in the body, if you don't use it, you lose it. Rotator cuff muscles can get torn from trauma, uneven stress from repetitive motions, or just wear and tear over time. There are several ways to strengthen your rotator cuff muscles so your shoulder will be able to handle increased stress without compromising the muscles themselves. You can perform the following exercises to protect yourself from future rotator cuff injury:

External Rotation with a Resistance Band

Tie one end of the band to a stable surface and stand perpendicular to the band. With the hand furthest from the surface, hold on to the band and keep the forearm parallel to the floor. Press a towel between your elbow and ribs. The anchor point of the stable surface should be pulling your hand toward the chest. With your palm facing inwards and a neutral wrist, rotate the shoulder and bring your knuckles to the outside of your body.

Internal Rotation with a Resistance Band

Tie one end of the band to a stable surface and stand perpendicular to the band. With the hand closest to the surface, hold onto the band and keep the forearm parallel to the floor. Press a towel between your elbow and ribs. The anchor point of the stable surface should be pulling your hand away from the chest. With your palm facing inward and a neutral wrist, turn the shoulder and bring your knuckles to the inside of your body toward your belly button.

Rowing with a Resistance Band

Tie a band around a stable surface at chest level. Hold the two ends of the band with each hand and step back until you feel tension. With both hands, pull the band towards your body without arching the back.

Frozen shoulder

This condition is also called adhesive capsulitis and occurs when the shoulder capsule gets inflamed. Clients with frozen shoulder typically complain of pain and stiffness during shoulder movements and also have trouble sleeping.

Frozen shoulder progresses in three phases:

1. **Freezing phase**: all shoulder movement increases pain. Range of motion is severely limited.

2. **Frozen phase**: Stiffness in the shoulder remains but the pain decreases gradually

3. **Thawing phase:** pain keeps decreasing and range of motion improves

There are no known causes for frozen shoulder, but it is more common in females over 40 years old and people with thyroid issues or diabetes. One of the worst things you can do for frozen shoulder is leave it alone and not move it. The frozen shoulder joint is stiff already, so if you don't stretch it, then it will become even stiffer and harder to move. Some of the techniques we use at Next Level PT to break up frozen shoulder tightness are needleless acupuncture and manual therapy. These are both hands-on techniques that help to regain movement while decreasing pain at the same time. Some basic exercises we recommend when suffering with frozen shoulder are:

Pendulum

Hold onto a surface with the unaffected arm and bend forward slightly at the hips. Let the affected arm hang toward the floor. Stand in a lunge position. Rock your hips and feet forward and backward and let your hanging arm move freely in a circular motion. The affected arm should feel as if someone is pulling on it.

Finger Wall Walk

Facing a wall, reach out to touch the wall at waist level with the fingertips of the affected arm. With your elbow slightly bent, slowly walk your fingers up the wall until you've raised your arm as far as you comfortably can. Your fingers should be doing the work, not your shoulder muscles. Slowly lower the arm (with the assistance of the good arm) and repeat. As the shoulder becomes less inflamed and stiff, the range of motion will improve.

Towel Pull Up Stretch

Hold one end of a long towel behind your back and grab the opposite end with your other hand. Hold the towel in a vertical position. Use your good arm to pull the affected arm upward to stretch it. Hold the bottom of the towel with the affected arm and pull it toward the upper back with the unaffected arm.

Cross Chest Stretch

Use your good arm to lift your affected arm at the elbow and bring it up and across your body to the opposite shoulder. With the good arm, apply gentle pressure to stretch the affected shoulder. Hold the stretch for 30 to 60 seconds.

6 TIPS FOR NATURALLY EASING SHOULDER PAIN WITHOUT VISITING YOUR DOCTOR

Tip #1: Optimal Sleeping Positions

Approximately 70% of my shoulder patients complain about difficulty sleeping. That's too much!

Here are some tips for the way you sleep:

> **Back sleeper:** while laying on your back, place a small pillow or towel roll under your elbow to line up the shoulder with your body

> **Front sleeper:** this actually is a very stressful position for your neck, so it is generally advisable to sleep on your side or back. If you have to sleep on your stomach, place a small pillow or roll under your elbow to support the joint.

> **Side Sleeper:** hug a pillow with your top arm. Your top shoulder should be aligned with your torso. This is especially important for people suffering with rotator cuff tears and frozen shoulder.

Tip #2: Avoid Lifting in Weird Positions

Do you always reach behind you to grab something from the back seat of your car without turning around? Or try to lift a heavy grocery bag without bringing it close to your body? Stop doing that!

These actions put extra load on your shoulders in positions where it has minimal stability or strength, a perfect recipe for an injury. When it comes to lifting, make sure to do all the heavy lifting with your legs, not your back or arms. Your arms should serve to secure objects close to you so that your legs can do the hard work.

Next time you need to get something in the back seat, get out of the car to get to it. As for the groceries, drag it close to the edge and then lift with your legs. Leave the shoulders out of it!

Tip #3: Correct Your Posture

Remember when your mother told you to sit up straight? Sorry, but she was right!

The shoulders, like most joints, work best when they are in the proper alignment. Putting the shoulder in the best position for it to work ensures that your muscles do not strain when performing any motions.

When you slouch forward, the shoulder is rotated forward too, which makes lifting the arm more difficult. Your neck muscles and other muscles start trying to help when lifting your arm, which can eventually lead to shoulder or neck pain.

Test it out yourself. Try to lift your arm over your head while slouching. Then sit up straight and lift your arm again. You'll notice the difference in how much your muscles have to work.

Make it easier on your shoulders. Correct your posture to make sure the muscles moving your shoulder don't have extra work they can't handle. Mom will be proud!

Tip #4: Avoid Always Carrying Your Backpack or Bag on One Arm or in One Hand

For this, you're likely going to need to completely flip everything you've done for years when it comes to carrying bags.

Carrying a work bag or even shopping bag over one shoulder means that the weight is not evenly distributed. The result is that one side of your body is under more pressure than the other. Guess what happens to the side of your body carrying the extra weight all these years? It's likely to be the side where you're feeling the pain and tension most.

Worse, if you carry the bag over one shoulder all the time, you could end up with a curvature of your spine. That would cause tension and pain, too, not to mention a funny-looking and unhealthy posture.

Tip #5: Avoid Sitting for More Than 20 Minutes at a Time

There's so much gossip that surrounds shoulder pain. But this is a FACT: you and I were not designed to sit. It goes against every basic, fundamental rule of the way we originally evolved as humans. When you sit, approximately 10x more pressure pushes down on your spine from your head than when you stand tall. That's a lot of extra pain and tension in the shoulder region. It's because most of us slouch, or flop, meaning that the muscles in your spine (called your core muscle group) that are designed to protect you just don't have a chance to work.

Tip #6: Stay Hydrated

One easy way is to cut out things that dehydrate you. These include coffee, tea, alcohol, and energy drinks. Being dehydrated can cause fatigue, dizziness, and muscle ache.

It's also important to keep water intake up to reduce unwanted tension in your neck and shoulder muscles. Drink water often during the day. Your shoulders will thank you for it.

CHAPTER 7

BACK PAIN

Have you ever lifted something heavy without thinking much of it and felt a pull in your back or shooting pain down your legs? Does your low back feel achy after sitting all day at work? We hear these complaints all the time from clients that come to Next Level PT for specialist back pain help. About 80% of adults experience low back pain at some point in their lifetimes. It is one of the most common reasons people take off work in the United States. The best part about back pain is that it's totally preventable in the first place!

This chapter will dive into common diagnoses our clients have when suffering with back pain. My goal is to give you awareness of what you can do to take stress off your back so you can decrease pain and prevent it from coming back.

BACK PAIN IS DIVERSE

The interesting thing about back pain is that two clients can complain of the same symptoms but have different causes. This is why your relative or co-worker's back pain exercises may not be right for your situation. There is no perfect back brace, exercise, or stretch that solves all back pain issues. At Next Level PT, one of the first things we teach you is to find patterns and recognize triggers for your back pain. As you gain awareness of how your body moves and what positions increase your back pain, we modify the plan to support faster recovery.

One of the main factors that affect back pain recovery is how long you have lived with it before seeking help. The acute back pain stage lasts up to three months and can occur when you suddenly feel a pull in your back while lifting or twisting. During this time, most people take it easy, pop a pain pill, or rub a little cream in to get some relief. These strategies might help temporarily, but they don't address the triggers and positions that caused your back pain in the first place. When your back is irritated already, it becomes more vulnerable to stress and additional flare ups.

If your back pain has not resolved after three months, it goes into the chronic stage. The difference between acute and chronic back pain is sort of like a paper cut. Imagine you have a paper cut between your thumb and the index finger. Every time you spread the index and thumb finger, you feel irritation on the cut. Common sense says that you would stop spreading those two fingers until the skin closed and healed properly. You might even put a bandaid on the cut with anti-bacterial ointment to prevent infections and speed up healing. Barring any unforeseen circumstances, your cut would heal completely and there would be no more problems moving your fingers.

This is the equivalent of finding the position that adds stress to your back and not triggering it. But imagine you kept spreading the thumb and index finger because you weren't conscious of it or the paper cut pain didn't bother you enough, so you lived with it. Of course the paper cut would keep re-opening and delay healing.

Fortunately, this means that whether you have acute or chronic back pain, most cases can be solved without the need for pills, injections, or surgery. Your body can self-heal when given the correct guidance and movement program.

WORDS MATTER MORE THAN YOU THINK

One of my PT mentors always told me that how you say something is more important than what you say. I'm always reminded of this whenever a new client calls my clinic or comes in for our free discovery session. Many times, we ask the person for their story, what have they tried, and what they've been told about their situation. It never ceases to amaze me how many healthcare professionals use negative language that puts fear, doubt, and worry into the client.

One recent client, Jay, is in his mid 40s and went to his doctor after hurting his low back lifting up his son. His physician took an x-ray and told Jay he had "the spine of an 80 year-old," "damage has been done," and "arthritis is in your future." Imagine your doctor telling you that. How would you feel? You would probably feel hopeless, terrified, or broken. Jay certainly did. In our experience, clients that have been exposed to negative language from medical professionals take longer to recover because they believe they can't get better or that there is nothing they can do to reverse the "damage" done.

Shortly after that, a chiropractor told Jay he had a disc bulge that would require weekly treatments. He was told not to bend forward or "lift anything over 20 pounds," otherwise it would put him at risk for back surgery. Fearful that he would need back surgery, Jay stopped picking up his son to play and relied more on his wife to do house chores and other tasks that require bending forward. His relationship with his family became more stressful. He was taking pain pills prescribed by his doctor and wearing a back brace from the chiropractor, but his back was getting increasingly achy every week. Over time, he only felt comfortable while wearing his back brace. This went on for 3 years before a colleague recommended he visit our clinic.

During our discovery session, Jay voiced his frustrations with the situation. He felt trapped. He wasn't able to enjoy family time because of the fear his back would get hurt and require surgery. When I explained what a disc bulge was and how it is a reversible injury, Jay was hopeful for the first time in a long while.

Jay had thought nothing could be done. After all, his doctor said he had "the spine of an 80 year old." So I explained to Jay the different phases of care at Next Level PT that he would need in order to get him from his current situation to a place where he would be able to bend forward without a brace and pick up objects over 20 pounds, like his son. Jay was skeptical but willing to try anything to avoid back surgery, play with his son, and enjoy family time again.

The key to Jay's recovery was starting with small steps. The first few weeks included very focused and specific education on how to activate the proper core muscles to protect the low back when bending forward. After Jay got better at this, I taught him how to bend from the hip as opposed to the low back. This is called a hip hinge and is one of the most important motions to learn for people who bend forward and put too much stress on the low back. Within 3 months, Jay went from being fearful of all bending motions to be able to tie his own shoes and pick up his son without increased back pain.

To Jay, I was a miracle worker, but he didn't realize that I see people like him every day of the week. Many people have been told by their doctors and healthcare professionals that nothing could be done or that they have to give up something for the rest of their life. As Jay's case shows, this is simply not true. If you've ever been told that nothing could be done for your situation or that you have to live with your aches and pains, contact us at **nextlevelpthouston@gmail.com.** We can develop a natural solution to get you back to living life on your terms.

X-RAYS OR MRIS DON'T DEFINE YOUR BACK PAIN

If you've ever visited your doctor for back pain, they've most likely sent you for an x-ray or MRI scan. This is a common way for physicians to rule out any structural and muscular issues. But what happens when both tests come back negative? You would probably be given a diagnosis of "non-specific back pain" and pain pills for several weeks.

This is exactly what happened to our client, Jason. He is 53 and has been suffering with back pain for years. He works as a construction manager and sits for 8 hours a day. His back pain would feel better with movement and get worse the longer he sat at his work desk. Twice a year, when the pain became excruciating, Jason would go to his doctor to get an x-ray or MRI done. The results always showed negative findings, so he would leave with another script for muscle relaxants. This cycle went on and on because he was being treated based solely off imaging.

The problem with x-rays and MRIs is that they are usually taken at the painful site. They don't take into account how the rest of the body or posture also affects that area. Back pain is commonly increased with different postures and movements. Until you figure out the cause and fix it, the symptoms will always be present. In Jason's case, he had a problem with his resting pelvis position during sitting. After several sessions of education on sitting positions, Jason's symptoms started to decrease. He no longer suffers with back pain during prolonged sitting. MRIs and x-rays alone won't show you the cause of back pain when there are movement and postural dysfunctions.

SURGERY SHOULD ALWAYS BE YOUR LAST RESORT

According to the Agency for Healthcare Research and Quality, 500,000 people get surgery for low back problems each year. However, a report by John Hopkins Medicine shows that fewer than 5 percent of people are good candidates for back surgery.

Many people who go under the knife for back problems weren't good candidates to begin with. It's no wonder that most people who get back surgery still have pain months or years later. The failure rate for back surgery is so high that there is a term for it, **FBSS (failed back surgery syndrome)**. There is no other equivalent term for any other type of surgery.

Back surgery can accomplish several things: relieve compression of a nerve, shave off bone spurs, or stabilize a joint. If the unstable joint or compressed nerve is a result of a movement or postural compensation, however, surgery will not fix the cause of the problem.

The 5% of people who are considered good candidates for back surgery present with symptoms such as:

1. Sudden bowel or bladder incontinence or progressive weakness in the legs. This is an emergency and can be a sign of cauda equina syndrome.

2. Severe, continuous abdominal and back pain. This can be indicative of abdominal aortic aneurysm and is also an emergency.

3. Broken bones or torn tissues as a result of trauma that requires stabilization

4. Radiating pain, numbness, or muscle atrophy for a period of at least 6 months that doesn't get better with conservative, non-surgical methods.

If these symptoms don't apply to your back pain, you are part of the 95% that aren't good candidates for surgery. And you should never get back surgery if you haven't tried conservative options such as physical therapy, chiropractic, acupuncture, and massage. Don't give up after one unsuccessful experience. It is imperative that you find a practitioner that specializes in working with back pain. If you went to a doctor who was not the right fit, you wouldn't stop going to all doctors.

Beware of companies that offer to view your x-rays or MRIs so they can offer you their surgery options WITHOUT assessing you. This means finding the triggers for your back pain. These can include a sitting or standing postural exam or a movement exam with walking or bending forward.

Finally, be very skeptical of "new" back pain treatments without scientific evidence or studies that show the success rate of the intervention.

SCAR TISSUE CAN MAKE A SUCCESSFUL BACK SURGERY GO BAD

In order to perform back surgery on the spine, a surgeon has to cut through the skin, myofascial system, and underlying structures. After surgery, the body creates thick, tough scar tissue on the myofascial system. In the early post-surgical stages, this scar tissue may have little effect on pain or stiffness in the body because the nerves, muscles, and blood vessels are still healing. As time passes, however, these structures heal and the scar tissue becomes thicker, thereby creating increased tightness on the whole fascial system. This can increase compression throughout the whole body as well as the surgical site. You can have a successful back surgery that removes your symptoms but still develop pain years later because scar tissue was never addressed. This is exactly what happened to our client, Dee.

Dee is in her mid 50s and suffered from back pain for over 15 years. She worked in retail and had to stand at least 6 hours a day. Over the years, she tried medications, injections, and multiple disciplines such as physical therapy, chiropractic, and massage. Nothing helped. The numbness and tingling in her legs got worse, so she opted for back surgery. Dee felt like a new person after surgery. She was able to walk, play with her grandkids, and work in her garden without leg pain or numbness. Life was good, or so she thought.

Three years later, Dee started to have recurring low back pain with numbness and tingling in the legs. She revisited her surgeon who told her the scar tissue from the previous surgery was compressing a nerve. He recommended surgery to remove the scar tissue. Dee knew that surgery would only temporarily get rid of her scar tissue symptoms because there is nothing stopping more scar tissue from developing if she undergoes another surgery.

Fortunately, Dee's daughter researched non-surgical scar tissue options and contacted our clinic's scar tissue specialist. After two weeks of scar tissue release treatment, Dee's leg pain and numbness went away. We then worked with Dee to improve her overall muscle strength to prepare her low back to handle increased stress over the course of the long workday. Three months after Dee came to Next Level PT, her back pain and scar tissue symptoms were no more. She is currently back to working, gardening, and playing with her grandkids without restrictions.

If you had previous back surgery and your symptoms came back months or years later, it could be caused by scar tissue.

SCIATICA

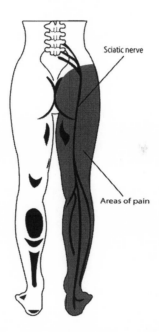

Sciatica is the term for any condition in which the sciatic nerve (the large nerve starting in your low back that travels down each leg) is compressed or irritated. These symptoms include feeling numbness, tingling, weakness, and pain in your buttocks, thigh, calf, and foot. Sciatica can result from a variety of reasons. In this section, we will dive into different diagnoses that can cause sciatica symptoms along with back pain.

One of the biggest factors in determining how quickly an individual recovers from sciatica is how long they wait to seek medical treatment.

Many times, people wait for it to get better or look for sciatica stretches on the internet without doing the proper testing to discover the cause of sciatica symptoms. It's important to know what the pain is and where it is coming from.

Disc Herniation

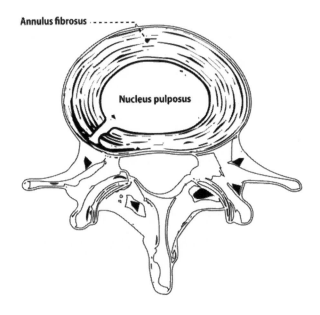

In between your spine bones is an intervertebral disc, which acts as a shock absorber. These intervertebral discs have 2 components: the annulus fibrosis (tough exterior) and nucleus pulposus (soft center). A herniated disc occurs when the nucleus pulposus pushes through the annulus fibrosis. Severe low back disc herniations can cause nerve irritation, particularly on the sciatic nerve. When this occurs, you'll feel numbness, tingling, weakness, or pain in your buttocks, thigh, calf, and foot. Pain can also increase in the legs when you cough, sneeze, or move your spine into certain positions. Think of the nerves as the wiring inside the wall that goes to a lightbulb (muscle). If the wiring (nerve) is compromised, then the flow of electricity (nerve conduction) is diminished going to the lightbulb. As a result, the light gets less electricity flow from the switch, so it flickers or is dim (tingling or pain).

Two Tests For Disc Herniation

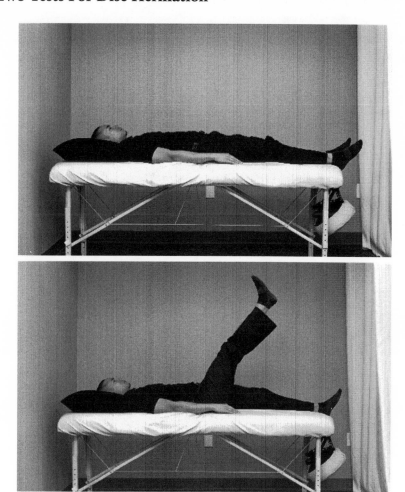

Straight Leg Raise

To perform this test, lie on your back with both legs straight. Lift one leg up toward the ceiling. If you have pain that shoots down your legs past the back of your knee, the test is positive for disc herniation.

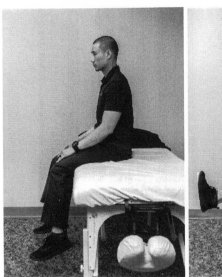
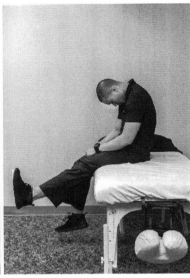

Seated Slump Test

Sit on the edge of a chair, straighten one leg, and bring your toes toward your nose. Round your back in a slouched position and look down toward your stomach. The test is positive for disc herniation if you feel an increase in symptoms of low back pain or shooting numbness and tingling below the knee down the legs.

Two ways to Stop Disc Herniation from Getting Worse

In order to prevent your disc herniation from progressing, you need to find out the direction of the herniation. It is always best practice to seek a medical professional to get assessed correctly. The most common type of disc herniation occurs when the disc moves too far back and to the side (posterolateral direction), pinching a nerve. Clients with this type of herniation typically present with increased symptoms while sitting, slouching forward, or leaning over to touch the toes. Symptoms decrease while standing or walking.

Prone Press Up

To perform the exercise, lie on your stomach with both elbows bent and your hands flat on the ground. Keep your back and hip muscles relaxed, and then use your arms to press your upper back and chest upward. Hold the press up position for 5 seconds before slowly returning to the starting position. Repeat this motion 10 times. Monitor your symptoms during each repetition. If your symptoms are moving toward the low back with each movement, that is a good sign.

If your symptoms are not changing or are increasing as you press up, you may need to try a less aggressive position called the stomach prone. For the stomach prone, lie flat on your stomach while doing the exercise and continue to monitor the symptoms. If stomach prone reduces the pain, numbness, and tingling symptoms, then perform several sets of 30 seconds in this position.

Standing Lumbar Extension

The great thing about the standing lumbar extension exercise is that can be done anywhere. Stand up tall with your feet shoulder-width apart. Place your hands on both sides of your hips. Slowly bend your spine backward as far as you can. Hold the end position for three seconds, and then return to the starting position. Be mindful to bend from the low back and not the knees. The most common mistake people make with this motion is bending from the knees so it seems like they are bending back further.

Repeat this exercise 10 times and monitor your symptoms with each movement. The intensity of the pain, numbness, tingling symptoms should decrease with each repetition. For best results, perform this exercise during the day after you've been sitting or bending forward for a prolonged period.

Lumbar Stenosis

Lumbar stenosis is a condition in which the spaces along the lumbar spine (low back) become narrow. This can be caused by disc bulges, degenerative changes, bone spurs, or arthritis. The symptoms are similar to those of disc herniations. One way to differentiate between disc herniation and lumbar stenosis is finding out which positions trigger your symptoms. Clients with lumbar stenosis typically are over age 55 and have increased numbness, tingling, or weakness in both lower extremities while standing or walking. Sitting or bending forward can temporarily help alleviate lumbar stenosis symptoms by opening the space that is compressing the nerve.

Lumbar Stenosis Test

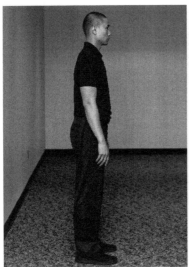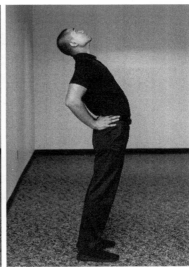

Standing Lumbar Extension

If you've read the treatment for posterolateral disc herniation, you should be familiar with this exercise. This movement can also be used as a test for lumbar stenosis. As you perform the standing lumbar extension, if you feel the back and leg symptoms increase and shoot past the knees, it can indicate lumbar stenosis.

As with most diagnoses discussed in this book, there is no one test that will definitively confirm you have stenosis. Think of a lawyer building a case. The more evidence the lawyer has that defends their client, the easier it is for the jury to reach a decision in their favor. Be sure to consult a healthcare professional who performs several tests to reach a diagnosis.

Two Exercises to Reduce Spinal Stenosis Symptoms:

Floor Reach Down

Sit on the edge of a chair with legs open wide. Bend forward and reach toward the floor with both hands. Perform this motion for 10 repetitions. On the last repetition, hold the downward position for 30 seconds. Monitor your symptoms during each movement for any changes. If symptoms moves toward your back, that is a good sign. If symptoms start increasing in intensity or shoot down the legs, stop the movement and return to the starting position.

Posterior Pelvic Tilt

Many people with lumbar stenosis present with an excessive lumbar lordosis posture (curved low back). This pelvic position increases compression to the low back and overstretches the abdominal muscles. The posterior pelvic tilt exercise helps bring the pelvis to a more favorable neutral position so that the low back can decompress and get relief.

In order to perform the pelvic tilt, lie on your back with both knees bent and feet on the floor. Put your hands on the side of your hips. Squeeze your butt and stomach muscles and use your hands to rotate your hips toward you. If you're performing this motion correctly, the low back arch should be flat against the floor. One way to check your pelvic position is by trying to place your hand underneath your low back. If you are performing the exercise correctly, your hand should not be able to fit underneath your back.

Another way to perform the posterior pelvic tilt is to imagine that your belly button is the barrel of a cannon. The cannon is attached to two handles on each side (both hips). The cannon can only be adjusted either toward your nose or toward your knees. When you are lying on your back with both knees bent, the belly button should be facing the ceiling. A posterior pelvic tilt movement is the equivalent of using your hands to rotate the hips upward and adjusting the belly button so that it is pointing towards the nose.

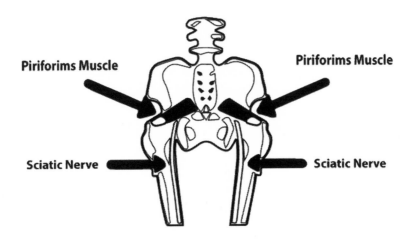

Piriformis Syndrome

The piriformis is a muscle that originates from both sides of the sacrum bone and attaches to the hip bones. In between this muscle runs the sciatic nerve. Piriformis syndrome occurs when the muscle tightens up and clamps down on the sciatic nerve. When this occurs, you can experience sciatica symptoms such as low back pain, hip pain, weakness, or tingling and numbness shooting down the legs. In most cases of piriformis syndrome, the symptoms are on one side of the body.

Piriformis Syndrome Test

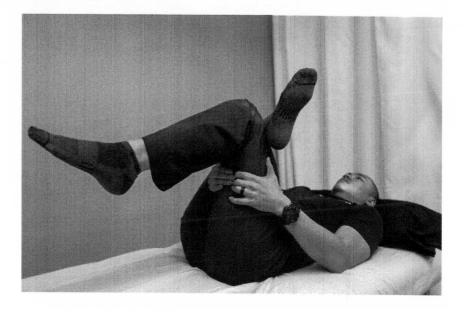

If you're currently experiencing the sciatica symptoms mentioned above, use this test to determine if the piriformis muscle is involved. Lie flat on your back with both knees bent. Take one leg and cross it over the opposite thigh. Let's say you cross your right leg over your left. The next step is to use both hands to pull the back of the left thigh toward your chest. You should feel a pull in the deep buttock of the right leg. Repeat this pull motion by switching the legs. If the buttock pull on one side of the body is more tender and triggers the sciatica symptoms, it is most likely that the piriformis muscle is involved on that side.

Two Exercises to Reduce Piriformis Syndrome Symptoms:

Golden Rules:

- Always test the left vs right motion
- One side should be more painful or tight while the other should feel normal
- Work the non-painful, normal side

- Re-test the original painful/tight side to see if there is any decrease in pain or improvement in ease of motion
- If working the good side improved the original painful/tight side, continue reworking the good side
- If your symptoms increase when testing both left and right sides of the body, stop working on that motion

Trunk Rotation Twist

Sit on the edge of a chair and rest both hands on your stomach. Turn your trunk to the left and repeat to the right. One side should feel more painful and/or restricted. If you can't differentiate between the sides, try breathing in and out while you do it. One side should feel more difficult to breathe.

Once you find the side that is less restrictive in terms of pain, breathing, or symptoms, perform trunk twists to that side in 2 sets of 20 repetitions. Retest the opposite side to feel whether the symptoms improved. If they did, repeat working 2 sets of 20 repetitions on the good side until the symptoms on the original tight and/or painful side disappear or stop getting better.

Piriformis Stretch Hold

This exercise is the same starting position as the piriformis test. If you performed the piriformis stretch test correctly, one side would have presented as more painful, tight or restricted. Perform a stretch and hold on to the good side for 60 seconds. Repeat this for three more times before retesting the symptomatic side. If the symptomatic side feels better, repeat several more rounds of stretching on the good side.

The reason why we don't initially work the tight or painful side is because that area is already irritated. If something is sensitive and painful, why would you want to pull and stretch on it? In many cases, that will only make matters worse.

Think of an arrowhead pointing upward toward the top of the page. On both sides of the arrowhead are a team of people playing tug of war with the rope attached to the apex of the arrowhead. The arrowhead will tip to whichever side pulls the hardest. When we perform the left vs. right testing, we are assessing which side is tighter or has more tension. If the right side has more tension and tightness the arrowhead apex tips toward the right. To restore balance, we need to pull more on the opposite side. When the body is balanced, the motions of the left and right side should both feel equal, and then the pain will decrease.

LIFT WITH YOUR LEGS, NOT WITH YOUR BACK

Have you ever bent over forward to pick up something and then felt your back tighten up or have pain? If so, you might be lifting with your back instead of your legs. The problem is most people are never trained properly on how to use their legs to take stress off the low back with lifting. Whether you're picking up light or heavy objects, you want to reinforce good habits.

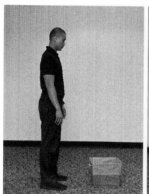 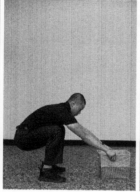 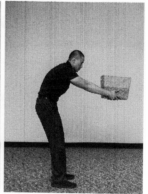

Can you spot what I'm doing above that is adding preventable stress to my lower back? For one, the box is too far away from my body. You wouldn't carry a heavy box with your arms outstretched instead of close to your body. Why work harder when you can work smarter? The second thing is that I'm rounding my low back and not putting my legs in a stable position to lift. Below are three ways you can position the body during lifts to take stress off the back and distribute it equally to the legs.

Squat lift

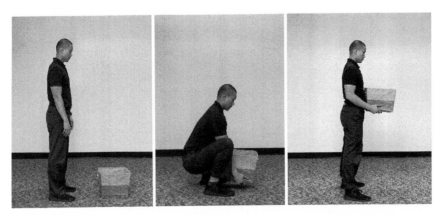

- Have a wide base of support. Your feet should be shoulder-width apart, with one foot slightly ahead of the other (most people use their dominant foot).

- Squat down toward the floor, bending at the hips and knees only. Your spine should not be rounded as you attempt this. If you have trouble, try putting one knee on the floor and your other knee in front of you, bent at a right angle (half kneeling position).

- Keep a neutral spine. Look straight ahead with your back straight, chest out, and your shoulders back. This helps keep your upper back straight and decreases extra stress to the low back.

- Hold the object as close to your body as possible and at the same level as your belly button.

- Slowly lift by straightening your hips and knees. Keep your back straight and don't twist or rotate as you stand up.

Hip Hinge lift

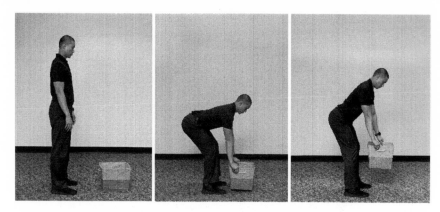

- Start by standing with your feet shoulder-width apart. Keep your chest up by standing tall.

- Shift your weight to your heels and move your hips back while bending them. Imagine that you're holding grocery bags with both arms and you're sticking the butt out to trying to close the car door behind you.

- Keep your chin down and your head in a neutral position as you are hinging. The goal is to keep your back straight while your chest moves toward the floor.

- Your torso should become more horizontal, and you should have a slight bend in the knees.

- Once you've reached the end position of the hip hinge, you should feel a stretch behind the legs. Keep your hands close to your body. There should be no back discomfort.

- Exhale while returning to your standing position. As your chest rises, bring your hips forward and squeeze your butt muscles at the top of the motion to complete the move.

Golfer's Lift

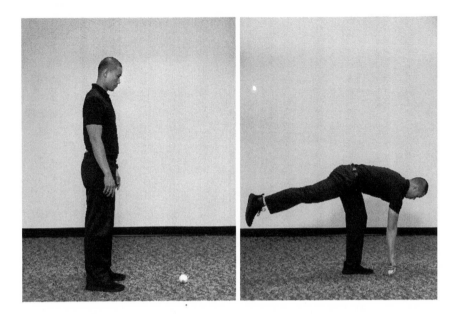

This movement is very useful to avoid excess stress to the back when lifting out of a bin or picking up small objects off the floor.

- Start by standing near the object to be picked up. Lean forward with a straight back while kicking back one leg. This acts as a counterbalance to the weight bearing leg.

- The opposite hip bends and the torso becomes almost parallel to the floor. One arm reaches to pick up the object while the other is often holding onto a stationary object for support.

- When done correctly, you will feel a stretch on the back of the weight bearing leg at the end position. Exhale when returning to your standing position.

7 QUICK TIPS TO RELIEVE BACK PAIN WITHOUT PAIN PILLS

Tip #1: Pressure Relief Sleeping Positions

Lie on your back with pillows under both knees. Make sure the pillows you use are firm enough not to flatten out over the course of the sleep cycle. Since your knees are raised higher than your hips, the pelvis rotates backwards and reduces pressure on your low back, providing relief during sleep.

If you sleep on your side, place a pillow between your knees and ankles and hug another pillow with your top arm. This will help keep your spine aligned and reduce stress on your low back.

Tip #2: Limit Wearing High Heels

Wearing high heels can create 25 times more pressure on your low back than wearing cushioned, supportive shoes. This happens because the body's center of gravity shifts forward, causing the pelvis to rotate forward and low back muscles to compress.

Over time, wearing high heels can shorten your leg muscles and cause a weak or stiff low back. Imagine how much relief you'd feel if you could take that stress off your back right now.

Tip #3: Avoid Stomach Sleeping

The stomach sleeping position is the fastest way to deal self-inflicted damage to your spine and low back. Avoid this position at all costs. It causes your spine to be twisted in all the wrong directions and will cause you to wake up with pain and stiffness.

Tip #4: Choose Proper Footwear

There are many footwear options out there today. Unfortunately, most of them will cause or add to your back pain.

Most footwear lack the proper support and cushioning for your feet. This will cause extra stress on your knees, hips, and back while walking. Well-fitted, cushioned shoes will be able to accept shock and can reduce your back pain.

Tip #5: Avoid The Cross-Legged Sitting Position

Your spine is not designed to withstand repetitive twisting or turning positions. When sitting in a cross-legged position, you are doing just that. The muscles in the spine/lower back become overstretched and weak. This can increase your vulnerability to injury.

Tip #6: Daily Low Back Exercise Rituals

You want to be sure that any exercises you perform are working for your condition; this is closely linked to visiting a good physical therapist.

A consistent routine of doing strengthening exercises and stretches to the spine can decrease back pain through your 40s, 50s, 60s, and beyond.

In the same way that you brush your teeth twice per day to keep them clean and healthy, you need to work on keeping your back healthy.

Tip #7: Microcurrent Point Stimulation (MPS)

MPS is one of the most effective interventions to eliminate pain and release scar tissue. MPS can relax muscles, calm the nervous system, and release endorphins, the body's natural painkillers.

At Next Level Physical Therapy, we offer MPS treatments to help patients manage pain, release scar adhesions, and relieve muscle tightness.

CHAPTER 8

KNEE PAIN

Having a painful knee can really limit your mobility and independence. After all, our knees allow us to stand, sit, walk, jump, and run. The knee joint is considered a hinge joint, much like a door hinge. The hinge is what allows a door to open and close, the equivalent of bending and straightening out your knee. Unfortunately, your knees can take a beating from overuse, sports, repetitive twisting motions, or general wear and tear. In this chapter, we'll discuss common diagnoses that contribute to knee pain and how to stop the problem from getting worse.

DO KNEE BRACES, INJECTIONS, OR SUPPLEMENTS WORK?

Have you ever seen a commercial showing someone with excruciating knee pain who had to stop running or exercising? Seconds later, they are wearing a knee brace and back to moving around without any issues.

The knee brace is one of the most commonly purchased accessories among our clients with knee pain. There is a time and a place for knee braces. The reason why people have less pain when wearing one is because it gives the joint extra stability and support.

Think back to the door hinge analogy. Imagine that the screws which fasten the door hinge to the door frame are loose and causing the hinge to shift more every time the door opens and closes. Over time, stress is put on the hinge to hold the door frame and door together. Let's say you put some tape on the hinge to hold it in the position where it should be. The door will open and close with less stress to the hinge and screws. The tape is synonymous with a knee brace. This can work short term, but the long-term fix is to tighten the screws so the hinge is back in the correct, solid position. Then you don't need the tape holding the hinge anymore. The long-term fix for most knee pain cases is to address the muscles that support the knee so that the knee joint itself doesn't take excess stress.

There are several situations where wearing a knee brace is warranted. The first is if you are ramping up activity and need the extra support temporarily. Make sure not to make a habit of wearing the knee brace continuously, though, otherwise the supporting knee muscles can get weaker over time. Another situation is after knee surgery. After the procedure, the surgeon might determine your knee should not be fully weight-bearing in order to speed up healing or that it requires a certain angle for several weeks before progressing to the next step.

The options for supplements that help joint pain is increasing every year. Some of the popular ones on the market that show promise are vitamin D, glucosamine and chondroitin sulfate, turmeric, omega-3, ginger, and SAMe (S-adenosyl-L-methionine). While nutrition and supplementation are very important to recovery, be mindful that they are not enough to fix knee pain on their own.

Most of the clients who come to us for knee pain have been through several rounds of pain medications before their doctors recommended knee injections. The most common injections for knee pain include Corticosteroid, Hyaluronic acid, Platelet-rich plasma, and Stem cell.

Corticosteroid injections are used to reduce inflammation in the joint. They can provide pain relief for 2-3 months. The negative side effects include tendon weakening, cartilage deterioration, increase in blood sugar levels, and nerve damage. As a result of these effects, doctors limit these injections to 3-4 times a year.

Hyaluronic acid is naturally produced in your body. The main purpose is to hold water that keeps your joint tissues lubricated. With conditions like knee osteoarthritis, hyaluronic acid injections are used to restore the joint's fluid property and improve shock absorption. Treatments can range from 1-3 injections and provide relief from 4-5 months up to 1 year.

Platelet-rich plasma (PRP) injections use your own blood and platelets to promote healing. Platelets contain growth factors and proteins that increase healing in soft tissues. Research shows that PRP injections can alter the immune response to help decrease inflammation.

Stem cells are extracted from bone marrow or fat and then injected into the knee joint with the hopes of developing cartilage cells, decreasing inflammation, or slow down cartilage degeneration to reduce pain.

Knee braces, injections, and supplements are used to reduce inflammation or pain. The problem is that inflammation and pain are symptoms. Until you find the true cause of the knee pain or inflammation, supplements, braces, and injections can only provide temporary relief.

THE IMPORTANCE OF FOOTWEAR AND ORTHOTICS

As I'm writing this chapter, we are in the summer season of Houston. The days are hot and humid, and everywhere I look people are wearing sandals and flip flops. Unfortunately, most people don't know that poor footwear can cause extra stress on the feet, which travels up the chain toward the knee. The heel of the ankle is the first point of contact with the ground while walking, so inadequate footwear support can lead to the knee twisting or rotating more than usual with each step.

If you have to wear sandals or flip flops, make sure they have adequate heel and arch support. Sizing also matters. If they are too big, you might have a tendency to bend the toes with every step for grip. This motion causes extra stress on the bottom of the foot and can eventually lead to foot pain.

Ladies, if you have knee pain, please reconsider wearing high heels for your next formal event or work day. High heels shift your body weight to the balls of your feet and knees, therefore increasing stress on those joints. If you're unable to get away from wearing heels, I would recommend you bring a pair of sneakers or flats to switch into whenever you can. Another negative effect of wearing heels for prolonged periods may include tight calves and increased pressure to the low back.

My favorite shoe stores measure your feet and make recommendations based on the findings. Everybody's feet are shaped differently, with various arches and heights, so it is imperative you get fitted for the next pair of shoes you buy.

Another recommendation I make to many of our clients is orthotics. Orthotics are great for people who need extra arch support or put too much pressure on certain parts of the foot. Remember, your feet and ankles are your foundation, so you want to make sure they have adequate support for the knee that is just above it.

Tips for Buying the Right Shoes:

- Shop for shoes during the afternoon and wear the socks that you'll most often wear with the shoes. Your feet expand during the day, so this will give you a better sense of the day-to-day footwear experience.

- Get both feet measured at the store. Your feet change in size and shape as you get older, so you might be surprised to find out one foot is a different size than the other.

- Examine the shoe soles for thickness. Notice the cushioning and the feeling as you walk around on soft and hard surfaces.

- Check the heel on the shoe for sturdiness. Your heel is the first point of contact with the floor. Too hard means you have a lot of impact to the heel. Too soft means your heel won't have adequate support on some surfaces.

- Look for arch support. Shoes for different occasions require varying arch supports. If you have flat feet, you may require additional arch support.

- Toe bend in the shoe is also important. If the shoe is very stiff and doesn't allow the toes to bend, the movement will come from somewhere else. This can lead to compensation and foot pain in the long run.

How Jacob Saved His Knees By Working On His Ankle Stability

Jacob battled knee pain for 10 years with endless rounds of medications and knee injections. He described it as "a rollercoaster ride when the pain medications and injections worked for a few months and then wore off." Jacob is a 48 year old supermarket manager with a life-long passion for martial arts and running. He developed knee pain after working long hours at the supermarket in combination with weekend karate and running sessions. He started having heel pain that woke him up at night and made walking feel like he was "stepping on glass."

When Jacob started treatment at Next Level Physical Therapy, he was consuming 4 pain medications a day and receiving quarterly knee injections. He tried knee braces and supplements, but nothing seemed to work. He had to be on his feet 10 hours and walk at least 6 miles a day for work. That's a ton of mileage accrued over the last 10 years. With our comprehensive movement screen, we found that Jacob had flat arches on both feet. Every time he walked or stood in one position, the knees would collapse toward each other. Over time this caused his knee muscles to compensate and take on extra stress.

We decided to start on Jacob's feet and ankles because they are the first point of contact with the ground when he stood or walked. Because of his flat arches and unsupportive footwear, his feet were unable to accept the weight and load with every step. His home exercise program included exercises to improve his arches and mobility drills to improve his range of motion.

Here's how to perform those exercises for yourself:

Arch up

Start with your feet flat on the floor. Lift your toes off the floor until the balls of your feet are pressing into the ground. Try to elevate your arch higher by pulling the heel and the bottom of the big toe together. Do this without turning your knee out.

Big Toe Flexion

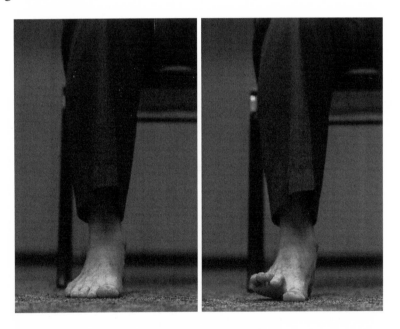

Keeping your heel and the balls of your foot on the floor, raise up all your toes. Then lower the big toe to the floor, keeping all other toes up.

Big Toe Extension

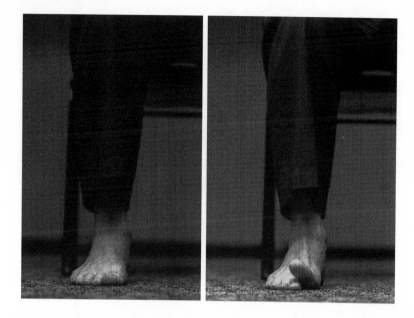

With your feet flat on the floor, raise your big toe while keeping all other toes, the balls of your foot, and your heel on the floor.

We also provided Jacob a program during his work break in order to take the stress off his recent foot pain. You can also try these massage and stretching techniques:

Foot Massage

Get a small firm rubber ball and roll your foot around on top of it. This will allow you to put some good pressure on specific points of the foot to give it a nice massage.

Freeze a water bottle and roll your foot back and forth on it. The cold will decrease pain and the rolling simulates a massage.

Use one or both of these ideas as needed based on the pain level in your foot. It is recommended to massage if you have tired feet or pain is present.

Big Toe Stretch

Sit with one foot flat on the floor. Bring the other foot to rest on the thigh. Using the fingers, gently stretch the big toe up, down, and to the side. Hold each position for 10 seconds. Repeat this 5 times before doing the same to the other foot.

Achilles and Calf Stretch

Face a wall and place both palms flat against the wall. Place one foot back, keeping the back leg knee straight. Both legs should be shoulder width apart. Now bend the knee of the front leg. Keep both heels flat on the floor and shift the weight of your hips forward until you feel the Achilles tendon and calf muscles stretching. Hold for 30 to 60 seconds before switching legs. Repeat two times on each side. For a more aggressive Achilles tendon stretch, bend the back knee as you shift the weight of your hips forward.

Jacob worked on his foot mobility and strengthening program diligently, which allowed him to eliminate his heel pain after only 5 weeks. His knee pain also decreased by 70% after each session. During the reassessment, Jacob's ankles stopped collapsing with each step and his knee was moving with less deviations. We continued to work on his ankle stability and strength by using resistance bands and balancing on foam surfaces. After 10 weeks of rehab, Jacob no longer had knee pain and was finally free of pain medications.

Here are the exercises that helped him build strength:

Ankle Eversion

Sit on the floor with both legs straight. Hold a resistance band and loop the band around the outside of your affected foot. If that is your right foot, for instance, press your left foot against the top of the band. Keeping your right leg straight, slowly push the outside of your right foot outward against the band and away from your other foot without letting your right leg rotate. The motion should only be coming from the ankle. Slowly come back to the starting position.

Ankle Inversion

Sit on the floor with your good leg crossed over your affected leg. Loop an exercise band around the inside of your affected foot. If that is your right foot, press your left foot against the top of the band. Keeping both legs crossed, slowly push the inside of your right foot against the band so that it moves away from your left foot. The motion should only be coming from the ankle. Slowly relax into the starting position.

Ankle Dorsiflexion

Tie the ends of an exercise band together to form a circular loop. Attach one end of the loop to a secure object or have someone hold it to provide resistance. While sitting on a flat surface, loop the other end of the band over the top of your affected foot. Keeping your knee and leg straight, slowly bend your ankle toward your torso to pull back on the exercise band. You should feel the shin muscles working.

Calf Raises

Stand with both feet shoulder width apart and keep both knees straight. Raise the heels of both feet as high as you can, then lower them back to the starting position. It is an up and down motion, not a back and forth rocking motion on the heels.

If you would like more information about foot and ankle pain, visit **www. nextlevelpthouston.com/foot-ankle-pain** to download "**The 6 Essential Tips To Reduce Foot And Ankle Pain In 14 Days.**"

MENISCUS TEARS AND KNEE SURGERY

Many of the clients we see with knee pain have meniscus tears or have been diagnosed with "bone-on-bone" arthritis. Their surgeons often say that their only option is knee surgery. However, a New England Journal Of Medicine study examined two groups of people with knee osteoarthritis and meniscus tears. One group underwent meniscus surgery while the other went to physical therapy. At the end of 6 and 12 months, the participants were tested for pain and physical function. Results showed no significant differences between the two groups.

The meniscus is cartilage that cushions the area between the thigh bone and shin bone. The most common way to stress the meniscus is bending and twisting the knee. Symptoms of a torn meniscus include swelling, stiffness, and pain around the knee. Many people also report the knee catching and locking with movement. Two of the most common orthopedic tests for meniscus tears are the Mcmurray's and Thessaly test. You will need a partner for both these.

Mcmurray Test

Lie on your back with the knee completely bent. The examiner holds your heel and rotates your shin bone inward, then straightens the knee while pushing the inside of the knee toward the outside of the knee. If there is a clicking sound that is accompanied by pain, it is a positive test for lateral meniscus issue.

In order to test the medial meniscus, you're in the starting position as before. The examiner holds your heel and rotates your shin bone outward, then straightens the knee while pushing the outside of the knee toward the inside of the knee. If there is a clicking sound that is accompanied by pain, it is a positive test for a medial meniscus issue.

Thessaly Test

Stand on one leg while the examiner provides his or her hands for balance. Bend your knee to 20 degrees and rotate the thigh on to the left and right three times while maintaining the standing knee 20 degrees bent. Be sure to test the good leg first and then the injured leg for comparison. The test is considered positive for a meniscus tear if the patient experiences clicking, catching, or locking on the bent knee.

If you tested positive for meniscus injury, I recommend you visit your orthopedic doctor for confirmation. The first rehab phase of meniscus injury is controlling the swelling and engaging the muscles around the knee to protect the meniscus from further damage. Some early rehab exercises include:

Straight Leg Raise

Lie on your back with your hips shoulder-width apart and your legs lying comfortably on a flat surface. Bend the knee of your non-affected leg at a 90-degree angle, planting your foot flat on the surface. Keep the affected leg straight and squeeze your thigh muscles. Lift the straight leg and hold 3 seconds at the top of the motion. Lower the leg to the floor with control. You should feel tension in the hip, thigh, and stomach muscles.

Supine Wall Slides

Lie flat on your back with both knees bent. Put the heel of the affected knee on a wall. Allow gravity to slide the heel down the wall without pain. Use the good foot to push the affected leg to a straight position. Repeat this motion.

Whether you've had a meniscus tear or have been diagnosed with "bone-on-bone" knee arthritis, there are more conservative options than surgery. Many times, a customized physical therapy rehab program can help decrease knee pain to the point where surgery can be avoided. This was the case with our client, Tabby. She was told by her surgeon that she had the knees of an 80-year-old and only surgery would take away her pain.

THE HIPS DON'T LIE

Tabby was 55 years old when she came to our clinic for chronic knee pain. She was depressed that the knee pain stopped her from playing tennis and spending quality time with her grandkids. The pain would wake her up during the middle of the night, walking became so difficult that she used a cane, and she would lean on the grocery carts when standing in line at the supermarket. She was desperate for answers and was scared of ending up in a wheelchair and losing her mobility and independence. During her 30s, Tabby had a meniscus and ACL surgery on her left knee. The orthopedic doctor told her another surgery was the only option if she wanted to decrease her knee pain.

Tabby was no stranger to looking for professional help. Over the past 10 years, she'd been to several doctors who recommended cortisone injections, pain pills, or different knee braces. None of it worked. She also tried chiropractors, massage therapists, and physical therapists. Worse yet, the last physical therapist only saw her for 15 minutes each session before giving her a sheet of exercises to do on her own in the gym and at home. Half the time, Tabby didn't know whether she was performing the motions correctly or not. She ended up quitting physical therapy after 3 weeks due to frustration and googling alternative solutions instead. She requested a phone call with us after seeing a video testimonial on a client we helped just like her. She wanted to know what her options were and decided to come in for a free consultation, which we call a discovery session.

During the discovery session, Tabby told me about the knee pain stopping her from playing tennis, sleeping, walking, or playing with her grandkids. She had surgery in her 30s and was determined to avoid further operations. Her greatest fear was losing her independence and even more quality time with her family and friends. After performing a movement screen on Tabby, it was obvious that her stiff and painful left knee caused her to limp and put excess pressure on other parts of the body. Further testing also revealed weak left hip, thigh and glute muscles that weren't working cohesively. In spite of these findings, Tabby had some things going for her: she was willing to try something different and was determined to find a natural solution to her knee pain without further medications, injections, or surgery.

At the evaluation, we created a customized program for Tabby's lifestyle. In order for Tabby to have less pain, we needed to loosen up her joints and get her leg muscles working together as one unit again. We did this by performing specialized, hands-on work to improve knee flexibility as well as specifically targeted movements to engage her thighs, glutes, and hips.

Here are 4 exercises that we taught Tabby during the transformation phase that can engage her glute and hip muscles to take stress off the knee:

Prone Heel Squeezes

Used to engage your glute (butt) muscles. Lie on the floor on your stomach. Put your chin on your hands, elbows out to the sides. Place your knees wider than your hips. Keep a folded pillow between your ankles and bend your knees so they are vertically pointing towards the floor. Squeeze the pillow with the inside of your feet and relax. You should feel the glute (butt) muscles engage.

Side-lying Hip Abduction Holds

Used to build hip muscle endurance. Lie on your side on a flat surface with your legs and feet straight and stacked on top of each other. Hold your lower arm bent and positioned under your head for neck support. Rest the upper arm on your upper hip. Raise the upper leg off the lower leg while keeping the knee straight and the foot in a neutral position. Continue raising the leg until you feel tension develop on the side of the top hip muscle. Hold this position for up to 60 seconds. As time passes you might feel a burning sensation in the top hip. You shouldn't feel the low back or groin muscles working or pulling. If you do, adjust your starting leg or body position. Slowly return your raised leg to your starting position in a controlled manner. Repeat this motion on both sides.

Fire Hydrants

Used to strengthen hip and glute muscles. Start with both your hands and knees on a flat surface. Place your shoulders above your hands and your hips above your knees. Tighten your core muscles and look down toward the floor. Lift your left knee away from your body toward the side. Keep your knee at 90 degrees. Hold this position for up to 60 seconds. Repeat this motion with the opposite knee. When performing this exercise, imagine a dog lifting the back leg to urinate on a fire hydrant. You will feel the glute and hip muscles working as you hold the top position. You shouldn't feel the low back during the motion.

Frog Pumps

Used to isolate the glute muscle activation. Place the bottoms of your feet together with your knees rotated out. Your feet should be about a foot or two away from your buttocks. Put your elbows firmly on the ground on both sides of your torso to stabilize your trunk. Press the hips up toward the air by squeezing the glute muscles. Squeeze and maintain the glute contraction at the top and then lower back down to the starting position. You should feel both hip muscles working. The low back shouldn't be arched or tightening up when performing this exercise.

As the weeks passed, Tabby's knees were less stiff and painful. She was able to walk and stand for longer periods of time. Her confidence started to grow and her mood improved. Next, we started phase 4, which is known as the transformation cycle. During this period, we taught Tabby how to maintain all the gains she made as well as use her own muscles and joints to regain movement she lost from the pain. This was a phase that Tabby never went through at her previous PT clinic. Unfortunately, most in-network PT clinics stop at the pain relief stage and never teach their clients how to get out of pain themselves so they can return to activities that they love. This leads to clients only getting short term pain relief and having to return to PT months later wondering why the pain came back.

The total rehab process took Tabby 4 months. Was it an easy process? Nope. Was the work required worth it to avoid another 10 years of knee pain and missing quality time with family and friends? Yes. Tabby was committed and determined to complete the program even when she had a trip between our plan of care. With the guidance of a specialist PT and specific hands-on work, Tabby is now able to play tennis with her peers, walk without a limp, and chase after her grandkids without restrictions.

Are we able to guarantee results like this to everyone? Unfortunately, no. There are many different factors that might affect someone's prognosis. That is why we offer a free discovery session to see if we can help you resolve your knee issues. If we are unable to help, we will gladly refer you to someone who can.

In order to see the 5 phases of the Next Level Physical Therapy process, turn to the back of the book. The time required in each phase is determined on a case-by-case basis.

The first start to any comprehensive knee program is taking stress off the joints. Here are two tips I use regularly with clients before getting into the hands-on treatment:

Be Selective of Where You Walk

Being selective of the surface that you walk on is an easy way to help knee pain. For example, walking on hard, uneven, or gravelly surfaces is going to make your knee pain worse. In contrast, walking on grass or on the sand means you'll suffer less because the surface is so much softer and kinder to all your joints. Even walking on a treadmill is nicer and healthier than hard concrete or pavement.

Weight Loss

Every 1-pound decrease in weight results in 4 pounds less strain on the body. So, if you drop 10 pounds, that equates to taking 40 pounds off your aching knees.

Let's think about this for just a minute. What is your goal weight? How can you achieve it? How much better might your body feel if you can reach that goal weight?

Weight loss is all about calories burned vs. calories consumed. Look to reduce your calorie intake by just 500 per day. That is exchanging one unhealthy snack or drink for water. 500 calories per day equals 1 pound per week. Combine a small reduction in calories with exercise and it'll become even easier to shed some pounds.

CHAPTER 9

YOUR INSURANCE MAY BE RUINING YOUR HEALTH

When was the last time you went to a doctor's office because of pain or sickness? Did the doctor spend time with you? Or did they simply ask what's wrong, give you a prescription while typing on their computer, and leave before you had a chance to ask any questions?

Unfortunately, this is a common experience for our clients who visit a traditional insurance-based clinic. There is a dirty secret your health insurance is not telling you. Every year, your health insurance premiums increase while the amount of money insurance companies pay your doctor or PT decreases. It is not uncommon for people to have $60 copays and high deductible plans that are thousands of dollars, which means they are still paying out of pocket for treatment even with proper insurance coverage. Often times, the **BEST** financial option for most people is to pay up front for their treatment plan and then submit to their insurance for reimbursement. The benefit of the fee for service treatment plans are that there are no hidden fees to the consumer and insurance is not allowed to dictate how the physical therapist can treat the client.

It used to be that physical therapists would see a patient, send a bill to the insurance, and get paid for the full amount. This allowed the PT to take time to hear the client's problems and form a comprehensive game plan without having to service several clients simultaneously. In the 1970s, the HMO (Health Maintenance Organization) was established, and it disrupted the insurance healthcare model. Health Insurance companies started to pay physical therapists a percentage of what was billed per session. As insurance reimbursed less each year, doctors and PTs were forced to see more volume of clients to make enough profit to pay overhead and salary.

When the volume of clients increases, the time spent with each patient decreases. This can lead to a rushed evaluation and treatment, creating subpar outcomes. An ideal physical therapy session would include an hour of one-on-one time to hear the client's story and figure out the root cause of their problems. If I were forced to see two to four patients an hour because of poor insurance reimbursements, it would be extremely difficult to find and treat the cause of the symptoms. We all know by now that treating symptoms might get temporary, short-term relief, but fixing the root cause will lead to full resolution of your problems. Insurance companies pay PTs differently depending on what treatment they bill for. From a business standpoint, many insurance-based PT clinics encourage their PTs to always bill and perform the highest-paying interventions regardless of whether the client needs it.

That's not the worst of it. Most insurance-based PT clinics only allow their PTs to see each client for 15 minutes before delegating them to a tech or aide to finish off the session. Have you experienced this type of facility, where everybody gets the same type of treatment whether or not their problem is the same? If you are using your insurance to pay for physical therapy, you could be subjected to only 15 minutes with your therapist. Fortunately for you, Next Level Physical Therapy mandates an hour evaluation for all our clients. We understand that some of you have previously been to a physical therapy office where you felt like you were just a transaction or were given a sheet of exercises to do on your own and then rushed out of the office.

At Next Level PT, we want to get to know and hear your story before you ever commit to any financial contribution to your treatment. That is why we offer a free discovery visit to our potential clients to make sure we can help them and to address their questions and concerns. To book your discovery session, visit www.nextlevelpthouston.com/discovery-visit

HOW MUCH DO YOU VALUE YOUR HEALTH?

To me, great health is priceless. Money can't flip a switch to make you healthy or take all your pain away magically, but it can provide you opportunities to seek the best specialists. Through all my years as a clinician, I have never heard of a patient bragging, "I got the cheapest provider to help me with my problem." My most successful clients always seek the best specialist to correct their problems and regain their quality of life.

Lauren came to see me after wasting months at a traditional insurance-based "PT mill" clinic. A PT mill is a clinic where they try to get as many people through the door while exhausting their PT insurance benefits without care for patient's progress. These clinics make money through volume of clients and not through high quality of care. She was referred to this clinic from her orthopedic surgeon, so she didn't think much of it and didn't do additional research. This was where she went wrong.

After several weeks at the PT mill, Lauren noticed that patients with different ailments were given the same type of treatment. Lauren had low back pain from previous surgeries and was put on the same machines as a client with shoulder pain. Her sessions with the PT were identical each time. She would pedal on the bike and then was given a heat pack for 15 minutes. After the heat pack, the PT gave her a 15-minute back massage, and then handed her a sheet of exercises to do on her own in the gym area.

After 3 weeks, Lauren's back pain was not improving, so she asked her PT, "Why does everyone get the bike, heat pack, massage, and self-exercise routine regardless of their diagnosis?" The PT replied, "That is just how we do things around here." Each session, Lauren would only get 15 minutes of PT and patient contact time before doing exercises without guidance. Half the time, she had no idea whether she was doing the exercises properly and felt that she was bothering her PT if she asked him to show her, since he was busy seeing 4 patients an hour.

When Lauren went back to her surgeon, he told her that since PT didn't work, injection or surgery was the next option. She immediately had an emotional breakdown. She'd been down this road before. The reason why she currently had low back pain was because of a previous back surgery. She'd gone to a similar PT clinic in the past and had no results, eventually opting for surgery.

Lauren was scared. She felt stuck and didn't want another surgery. Fortunately, she was in a mom's walking group where they often discuss healthcare and the issues they are facing. After sharing her PT experience, one of the moms told Lauren about Next Level Physical Therapy and how we helped her with low back pain. Lauren was skeptical when she called my office, but I understood that she has been duped by her previous PT clinic. This is a story I hear every day from potential clients all over town. After our phone conversation, I knew I could help Lauren, so I invited her for a free discovery visit to address her questions and concerns.

Lauren felt that the PT she previously worked with had good intentions but that she was a complicated case and needed more one-on-one guidance, especially exercising with the correct form. At our therapy evaluation, we worked together for a full hour to find the root cause of her low back pain and set up a game plan to address it. For the first time, she felt relief knowing that there was actually something she could do other than surgery.

During each one-hour session, we assessed and reassessed to make sure she was on the right path to recovery. Instead of handouts, we used Lauren's phone to record her performing the exercises to make sure she has the proper guidance to do them correctly.

It took 4 weeks of specialist PT to get rid of Lauren's back pain. She went back to her surgeon, and he was surprised at her recovery. She explained how the PT clinic he sent her to had a "cookie cutter" approach and gave everybody the same program. As a result, there were no improvements. Next Level Physical Therapy created customized treatments for her specific needs. This led to her speedy recovery.

CHAPTER 10

HOW TO FIND THE BEST PHYSICAL THERAPIST FOR YOUR NEEDS

E very industry has good and bad apples. What do you do when you go to a doctor's office and realize you don't get along with the doctor or the staff? Or worse yet, when after a few months of treatment your condition has not improved? You would probably get a second opinion from another doctor. There are so many physical therapy clinics, all claiming to do similar things, that it can be confusing to decide which one to go to. You wouldn't purchase a car without doing research and test driving it, so you should treat choosing your physical therapist the same. After all, your health is more important than your car.

As a consumer, you always have the choice of which physical therapy clinic you go to. You might get recommendations from your friends, doctors, or an insurance company website. Unfortunately, not all doctors have your best interest in mind when referring to physical therapy. Some doctors have a financial relationship with a therapy clinic and send most of their patients there regardless of whether the physical therapists working there are specialists in helping with your specific diagnosis. Next time your doctor refers you to physical therapy, do your own research to see if the therapists at the clinic are specialists in helping people with your ailments. Or your friend might refer you to a clinic that helped them with their problems, but your injury and goals may be different from theirs. Your personal preferences might differ from your friend's as well. They might prefer a quiet intimate clinic where you'd find comfort in a clinic where there is a lot of activity and upbeat music.

It is highly recommended that you call or visit the physical therapy clinic that you are considering to talk to the physical therapist that you would potentially be paired with for treatment. Pay attention to how much time the therapist gives you to listen to your story, address your concerns, and answer your questions before any financial commitment. How you do one thing is how you do everything. Clinics not allowing their therapists to give time to potential clients might be a reflection of how they treat clients during the whole treatment plan.

One of the unique things we offer at Next Level PT are free phone consultations for people to discuss their story and address any questions or concerns. This allows us to give more information to people so they can make the best decision for their health. For those individuals who have never experienced PT before or have been burned by other healthcare professionals promising results, we offer a free in-office discovery session. This allows you to discover how Next Level PT is different and determine whether we are a good fit to work together.

FIND SOMEONE WHOSE TREATMENT IS PERSON-FOCUSED, NOT DIAGNOSIS-FOCUSED

Often times in the healthcare world, people are treated as a transaction and not as a person. How many times have you called a doctor's office only to be asked for your name, date of birth, and insurance information instead of having a conversation about your health? You want a physical therapist who can spend time with you and explain your situation in a language you can understand. You should also want someone you can feel comfortable talking to about your needs and goals in order to formulate the right game plan for your treatment.

SEEK A SPECIALIST PHYSICAL THERAPIST FOR YOUR INJURY

Would you go to a family doctor when you have an orthopedic issue? Probably not. You would go to an orthopedist, who might refer you to a surgeon if necessary. This same concept applies when looking for the next physical therapist for your condition. Seek a physical therapist who specializes in helping people your age and with your condition. It is more likely they will get you back to doing things that you love faster, because they see people like you every day.

Questions to Ask a PT Clinic:

1. What specializations do your physical therapists have?

    Next Level PT: We have certified pain specialists, a concussion specialist, a scar tissue specialist, and exercise experts for aging adults.

2. What is the type of clientele you normally serve?

    Next Level PT: Most of our clients are age 50+ who are dealing with pain and want to get out of the vicious cycle of relying on pain medications, injections, and unnecessary surgery so they can return to doing activities that they love.

3. How many patients do the physical therapist see every hour?

    Next Level PT: We see one patient per hour unless the client requests otherwise.

4. How much one-on-one time do I get to spend with the therapist every session?

    Next Level PT: We spend 60 minutes of one-on-one time with the client throughout the whole session to ensure all questions and concerns are addressed

5. How can I contact my therapist after clinic hours and when can I expect an answer from them?

    Next Level PT: We have a text message system for our clients to contact us 24 hours a day and 7 days a week. Your therapist will get back to you within 24-48 hours to answer your questions and concerns. Communication is huge for us, and we never want our clients to feel they are on this journey to better health alone.

CHAPTER 11

THE BIGGEST MISTAKES PEOPLE MAKE ABOUT THEIR HEALTH

Getting stuck and frustrated is one of the most common things I hear from people suffering from neck, shoulder, back, knee, or foot pain. How long have you been stuck taking the same medicine or seeing the same providers and getting lackluster results? How would you feel if you could stop taking pain medications, skip another injection, or avoid surgery?

Here are some common objections I hear from people who are stuck and frustrated by neck, shoulder, back, knee, or foot problems:

I Want To Try To Get Better On My Own

Are you not ready to see a professional for your pain yet? Or do you not trust healthcare professionals because the last one you saw did more harm than good? Whatever the case may be, home remedies such as essential oils and creams do work with mild aches and pain. Unfortunately, it never fully relieves the issue for most people. Why wait several months or years of using the same methods with minimal results when you can seek specialist physical therapy help right now. At Next Level PT, we often help people who either got stuck trying to get better by themselves or have gotten worse with doing exercises they found online.

Samantha first called my clinic when she read one of my blogs on back pain. She told me that she'd had back pain for 27 years and had tried "everything under the sun," such as chiropractors, massages, physical therapists, injections, and back braces. Recently, she was introduced to a pain cream from her doctor that brought her pain down 20%. She said the back brace and cream made her pain more manageable, but she wanted to "feel normal and walk her dogs without having to use the brace."

When offered a free in-office consultation, Samantha said she would wait and try to get better on her own. Fast forward 6 months and we get another call from Samantha, distraught and in more back pain than ever. Her back brace, creams, and internet exercises no longer worked for her. She felt hopeless and frustrated. Fortunately for Samantha, we see patients with her issues daily, so we were able to get her into a free discovery session the same week and figure out the root cause of the pain during a movement screen. We created a customized plan to get her out of pain and back to walking her dogs.

My Pain Is Not Stopping Me From Doing Anything

When your pain is stagnant or slowly increasing over time, you might be able to get through the day as long as you take your time. You might still have the ability to get out of bed, take a shower, drive to work, and cook dinner at home. But you might have already stopped going to the gym or cut the time playing with your kids because it increases pain. This cycle can continue until the pain gets to a boiling point. Then it actually stops you from doing all the things that you love. The longer you wait, the more difficult it is and the longer it takes to help you get back on your feet. At Next Level PT, we specialize in helping people get unstuck from their current pain, and we also teach all of our clients how to prevent pain from coming back so that they can return to the activities that they love doing for as long as possible.

Joe called our clinic when he experienced increased back stiffness after a long day at work. The stiffness didn't stop Joe from working, but it made it more difficult to get out of the chair or play golf on the weekends. Joe worked a desk job and remembered how his father used to complain of back stiffness after sitting for prolonged periods. His father never sought a specialist PT to help with his stiff back, and one day he injured it playing golf. He never recovered and had to give up golf. Joe didn't want to have the same fate, so he came to Next Level PT for a mobility program to keep his low back loose and his golf game sharp.

It Is Too Expensive

How much would it cost if you weren't able to work because of the pain? How much would surgery and the rehab process cost? Can you put a monetary value on how your pain is affecting your quality of life and relationship with your family and friends? Could it be fear that you think physical therapy is needed for the rest of your life? All services at Next Level PT are customized and tailored to your individual needs to get you back to work or enjoying life as soon as possible. If several doctors determined that surgery was your only option for your condition, would you wait while your quality of life was decreasing every minute? Would your decision be any different if it were your parents or child in that situation? You certainly wouldn't be looking for the cheapest provider. You'd be searching for the clinic or person who specializes in their problem so they can give them the best possible chance for a full recovery.

I Want a Simple and Fast Solution

Think of all the times that you wanted to master a skill. It doesn't happen overnight. It requires time and effort. Getting your body away from pain so you can return to the activities you love requires the same. Most of the clients we help at Next Level PT have pain or imbalances in the body that developed over many years, so it will usually take more than one or two sessions to resolve the issue completely. What is the other alternative? Before finding Next Level PT, many of our clients took pain pills or received injections to temporarily numb the pain enough to deal with it throughout the day. This is a temporary solution to the problem, but it never fully solves the root cause of the pain. What if I told you that long-term intake of pain medications can cause organ failure? Would that change your mind of seeking a more natural solution? In order to get lasting results, you must master your body physically, mentally, and emotionally.

I Have No Time For Physical Therapy

Would you make time for physical therapy if I could guarantee that you will be out of pain and back to doing the activities that you love? Yes, you would. Unfortunately, I can't guarantee results, because there are so many outside factors beyond my control that can affect your prognosis. At Next Level PT, we can guarantee that if you give us your time, we will also commit our time to giving you more information about your health so that you can make the best decision going forward. This can take place during our free discovery session, where you tell us what you are going through, what you have tried, and what questions and concerns you have. We also understand that everybody's schedule is different, whether it's from a job or family commitments. This is one more reason why we create customized programs to not only cater to the time frame in which you want to get better but also consider how much time you have to work on yourself based on your schedule.

A client, Greg, came to us after his wife fell and needed surgery. Greg has been suffering from back pain for months and kept putting it off because of work and family demands. After his wife required surgery, he knew that he would need to spend more time as a caregiver. Fearing that his back pain would prevent him from caring for his wife and kids, Greg found Next Level PT online. From the start, he emphasized how little time he had available to work on himself. After all, he was working full time, doing house chores, and caring for his wife and kids. We created a game plan to fit Greg's hectic schedule. The key was also bringing his whole family into the session so we could strategize how everyone can work as a team to spread the load off Greg's shoulders.

As the family worked together, Greg found time to be consistent with his home exercise program and flourished. His back pain was gone in a few weeks, and he was able to care for his wife and kids without any setbacks.

After Greg was finished with physical therapy, he admitted, "I wished I would have listened to my wife and gone to physical therapy when I first got the back pain. Delaying treatment for my back limited how much I could care for my family in times of distress. Knowing what I do now, I have to make time to take care of myself in order to better support my family."

I'll Use the Internet to Help Instead

Thanks to advancements in technology and smartphones, we are more reliant than ever on the internet for answers. When was the last time you searched for that pain that you have been suffering with? You may have tried several home remedies or exercises that were listed as appropriate for your aches and pains.

Our client, Chris, found us online and came in for a consultation to find out about his chronic tight hamstrings and back pain. Chris was a hospital physician, so he consulted his orthopedic colleagues and did research online for months. When he came into our office, he was convinced he had hamstring syndrome. He complained of constant hamstring tightness regardless of movement or sitting. No matter how much he stretched, the muscles kept tightening up. The only temporary relief he got was when he took pain medications throughout the day. When I asked Chris what he was currently doing, he replied, "I'm doing several Youtube stretches for the hamstrings." He knew something was off when the back pain kept getting worse along with his hamstring tightness.

After performing the assessment on Chris, I found that he lacked hip mobility and that his glute muscles weren't activating correctly. This caused his hamstring to tighten up as a compensation strategy. Stretching the hamstrings was only treating the symptoms. He never addressed the cause of the problem. Chris realized that his assumptions of "hamstring syndrome" were incorrect.

The next time you are looking for health advice, please be wary of where you get your information. You can start by getting information from Google or WebMD, but it is always best practice to see a healthcare professional that is familiar with your condition, such as a back pain specialist PT. Fortunately for Chris, he came in before going through the vicious cycle of pain medications, injections, or surgery.

Another platform where most of our prospective clients learn exercises is Youtube. Personally, I love learning how to do things from Youtube, but exercises aren't one of them. The problem with Youtube is that there is so much information out there for the general public. If you do a search for back pain, there are thousands of videos showing different tips and exercises to do. It can get overwhelming trying to decide which video or exercise to follow. The issue is that the cause of back pain is different for everyone. Exercises are not a one-size-fits-all approach. Remember when Chris did Youtube stretches and the muscles got tighter? It's obvious that stretching was not helping the situation. During our consult, Chris showed me the Youtube video. The person demonstrating the hamstring stretch was in a position that added low back stress. It was no wonder his symptoms increased. Chris would have been better off seeing a specialist physical therapist and getting the proper exercises to move him along the road to recovery.

Most clinicians would get offended if a client came in telling them their self diagnosis and what treatments are needed based off of WebMd, Google, or YouTube. At Next Level Physical Therapy, we are ecstatic about that. It shows us that you value your health and are committed to getting better. But if you would like specialist help finding out why you're having aches and pains, contact us at **nextlevelpthouston@gmail.com**.

THE 32 FAQS OF PHYSICAL THERAPY

Q1. What is physical therapy?

Jack: Physical therapy is a proven strategy for easing the worries and concerns of people suffering from aches, pain, and stiffness, and then helping them move freely again, bending further, stretching more easily, and living an active and healthy lifestyle in their 40s, 50s, 60s, and beyond.

More, it lets people live free from the worry that the same problem will come back to haunt them anytime soon.

Q2. How long before I feel the difference from physical therapy?

Jack: There are two ways physical therapy can help. A good physical therapist will lift your concerns and ease your worries by telling you what's going wrong, often within 10-15 minutes.

Next, the speed at which the physical problem is eased is completely dependent upon your age, how long you've had it, how severe it is, and the treatment skills of the physical therapist. Rarely does anyone spend more than 3-5 weeks (unless suffering from chronic problems, severe injury, or surgical recovery) in our care before leaving happy. It often works that quickly.

Q3. Do I get personal support if I need it?

Jack: Yes. If you arrange to try PT with us, you'll be given almost full access to your therapist, who will be on hand to answer your calls, text messages, or emails for as long as you need.

Q4. Does PT help someone like me?

Jack: Here's a list of the types of people PT helps:

- **People aged 40+ who love to be active**
  Because men, women, and couples "on-the-go" have lots of good reasons to get better quickly

- **People still working (and who want to remain that way), especially sales people, managers, civil servants, engineers, office workers, teachers, manual workers, nurses, healthcare workers, lawyers, even doctors**
  Because they need to move easily and sit comfortably for long periods in order to perform well

- **People aged 55+ who are determined to remain independent**
  Because many people see the impact that poor physical health has taken on their parents

- **Especially active and involved grandparents**
  Because grandparents who play games with their grandkids, help with schoolwork, like to walk with them to and from school, take them places, or babysit them often tell us that's why they felt the need to come and try PT

- **People who take their health very seriously**
  Because many of the people who visit us are very proactive about their health. That means they read up on foods, vitamins, health topics, try to eat right, take vitamins or other supplements such as fish oil, and do their best to stay out of the doctor's office and

the hospital. The very same motivations to stay out of the doctor's office are the reasons why come to see a specialist PT like me.

Q5. What if I book an appointment today, but before I get to you, there's a positive change in my condition?

Jack: Great! That's the best outcome. Just give us a call to cancel your appointment. We just ask that you keep in touch to let us know how you're doing.

Q6. What should I wear to therapy?

Jack: Our office staff can tell you this on the phone. But you never have to remove large chunks of clothing. To make your PT experience as comfortable as possible, please keep in mind the location of your injured body part.

For example, if you have a lower back or shoulder injury, a loose top would be ideal. For a knee problem, please wear or bring shorts.

Patients will occasionally ask us if they can remove an item completely for ease or comfort of treatment. You are free to make that decision.

Q7. If I don't want to make another appointment after my first visit, do you take it personally?

Jack: Not at all. We know we can give you amazing care and results, but our first priority is to tell you what's going wrong and what would be your best options for care. Once we've done that, it is your decision on how you would like to handle your care.

Q8. How likely is it that physical therapy will be able to help me?

Jack: If your problem or concern is one of pain and or stiffness in the muscles or joints of the following area(s):

- Back
- Hip
- Knee
- Neck/Shoulder
- Ankle
- Foot/Ankle

Then it's 99% likely that PT will be able to help you in various ways.

Q9. Can I talk to a therapist before I book just to confirm PT right for me?

Jack: Absolutely. Just call us at **281-888-0047** or email your question to me at **nextlevelpthouston@gmail.com**

Q10. Will you do anything at the first session to help my pain?

Jack: Yes. It's always our intention to start making progress on the pain or stiffness immediately in addition to helping ease your concerns and frustrations.

Q11. Isn't PT just for young people who are injured and play sports?

Jack: Absolutely NOT. I'll be the first to admit that PT helps people who do play sports, but PT is actually much more valuable to help people over 50 who just want to stay active for as long as is possible.

Q12. Will I get any exercises to take home with me?

Jack: Only if the time is right and I think you doing them is not going to make your pain worse. However, I will give you as many hints or tips as possible that you can use when you go back home that night.

Q13. What will happen if I don't choose to go and see a physical therapist?

Jack: Your current predicament will continue, and you'll run the risk of doing unforeseen and untold damage to the joints if they're not moved back into the correct position or the muscles around them made stronger.

A failure to adhere to the right recovery program post injury could increase the risk of early onset arthritis in joints. 10 days is an important milestone. If pain and or stiffness are there at this point, they aren't going away on their own.

Q14. Something happened the other day, and now I'm in a lot of pain. How long should I wait before I see a physical therapist for help?

Jack: Don't wait! There will always be a number of ways we can help. Sometimes it's as simple as, "Do this, but don't do that..."

The first thing will be to tell you what **NOT** to do. So many people make fatal, uninformed mistakes when it comes to dealing with sudden pain. Every decision that you get wrong in the first few days will very likely add to the length of time it will take to get better.

Q15. Somebody mentioned a Chiropractor to me. What's the difference between a Physical Therapist and a Chiropractor?

Jack: To be brief, a PT looks for a cure. Our aim is to help you so much that you will not need to constantly keep coming back to us. So, a PT will work you out a plan to stop the injury from happening again.

We can perform some techniques very similar to osteopaths and chiropractors, such as manipulation of your spine, but we do added things such as massage and stretching and believe that the combination of that, plus exercises and posture correction, will first reduce your pain fast and also help you manage your pain in the coming years to avoid the need for repetitive visits to see us.

Osteopaths and chiropractors are both fantastically effective at reducing back pain, and many of the good ones will even refer their patients to a PT for services that they don't do.

Q16. I can't work this thing out. One minute I'm not bothered by it, the next it can quite literally take my breath away. Just when I think it's getting better, it hits me again! If I come in to see you when it's not hurting, will I be wasting my time?

Jack: No. Pain is not really what we do! Physical Therapy is about finding whatever it is that is causing the pain to happen in the first place. If your injury is a few weeks old, two things are likely to be happening. The first is that the joints and muscles are locked, stiff, or jammed in one place, so every time you get to a certain point they don't want to move and will give off a sharp pain. Second, you're likely to have tight and weak muscles. The combination of that plus locked joints equals long-term problems and increased pain

Q17. Is physical therapy guaranteed to help me like I hope?

Jack: There are no guarantees, as with most things in life. But, after a few sessions we will know whether physical therapy will be beneficial to your situation. We often have great success, but if there is an underlying cause that is not related to PT, we will do our best to refer you to someone who might be able to help.

Q18. Does this sort of thing happen to other people?

Jack: We see many people with the same sorts of injuries all day long, particularly within the 50-64+ age group who suffer from aches, pains, and stiffness.

Q19. What is the long-term benefit of choosing to see a physical therapist?

Jack: You have the freedom in your life to do what you want and when you want to do it, unrestricted by pain or stiffness.

Q20. How quickly will I be seen?

Jack: Our goal is to see everyone within a few days. We have often squeezed people in on the same day when needed.

Q21. I'm not in any pain per se. I'm just experiencing lots of stiffness and tightness, and I'm worried that something's about to go "pop." Am I right to consider physical therapy?

Jack: You are PERFECT for physical therapy (and us). Some people think that physical therapy is about ending pain, but that's only one thing we do. And it isn't even the best.

The aim is to stop you from ever getting to the point where you're in lots of pain by making your muscles flexible enough and your body strong enough to withstand the amount of activity you want to do, no matter your age.

Q22. What's the difference between a good physical therapist and a bad one?

Jack: four things

- The amount of "care" they take (this is easy to spot)
- The hands-on techniques and skills they use
- Their ability to accurately diagnose an injury
- How they communicate with you

Q23. Can physical therapy help me if I have arthritis?

Jack: Yes! Please understand that it can't CURE it, but it can very easily help manage the symptoms it causes. Many people come to therapy aged 50+ and suffering with "wear and tear" (arthritis) inside their knee joint, for example. We will minimize those aches and pains with a proper stretching and strengthening program.

Q24. I have had clicking, clunking, and cracking noises happening in my joints for a few years now. Now the pain is starting to get worse. I'm 48. Is physical therapy for me?

Jack: Yes. You're an almost perfect candidate for physical therapy. This is a common story. Most joint problems begin with warning signs like the clicks and cracks you've been hearing. A few years later, the pain starts. We can help prevent that.

Q25. I'm a cyclist, and I'm not in any pain on the outside of my knee when I rest, but it flares up whenever I get back on my bike. Is that common, and do I need physical therapy?

Jack: Yes and yes. Most sports injuries settle down so that you can walk around and do simple everyday things without pain. But as soon as you step it up a level or two, it lets you know in the way of tightness, pain, swelling, or stiffness.

Q26. Is there anyone that physical therapy ISN'T right for?

Jack: Yes. Anyone who is expecting a miracle and hoping to be fixed in one visit, which is rarely possible, particularly for injuries happening to men and women over 50.

Q27. What does physical therapy treatment actually entail?

Jack: Physical Therapy treatments can include things such as massage and manual therapy, stretching and loosening of joints and muscles, combined with exercises and advice to improve posture. We also have PTs who are trained in several specialized techniques and exercise programs, such as MPS Therapy, Concussion Therapy, LSVT BIG, and Total Motion Release.

Q28. Is physical therapy painful?

Jack: Not really. It is true that therapy is a very physical experience, so treatments may be a little uncomfortable at times, but we will always aim to be as gentle as possible and cause the least discomfort possible while getting your problem solved as quickly as we can.

Before we do any therapy techniques, we will tell you exactly what is about to happen, whether or not it is likely to hurt, and for how long.

Q29. Will I get any tips that I can be doing at home to help myself get better quicker?

Jack: Absolutely. The aim is to help you in every which way that we can, but you're only with us for an hour, so we aim to arm you with tools, hints, and tips that you can use to make a difference that you will feel, very quickly, on your own.

Q30. How important are exercises to my recovery?

Jack: Not as much as you may have been led to believe. They're more important in stopping the problem from coming back. They do play a role in your recovery, but most people do the wrong ones, at the wrong time, in the wrong order, for the wrong reasons. A good physical therapist will help you find the right exercises and create a program that works for you.

Q31. Do I need a referral from my doctor?

Jack: We are able to see anyone without a doctor referral for the initial consecutive 10 days. We would need a PT referral for the 11th visit and thereafter. Just give us a call and book. If you're willing to invest in your health, you're very welcome to come see us, and we would LOVE to take great care of you.

Q32. How often will I need treatment?

Jack: That is dependent upon the nature of your injury and how quickly you want the improvements. Our aim is to return you to full fitness and function as quickly and as safely as possible. Your PT will be in a better position to answer this following your initial consultation.

Big Tip: Getting in early nearly always means less time to recover and less physical therapy sessions needed.

HOW TO WORK WITH US

I hope you have gained knowledge and insight on ways to live healthier and to treat the cause rather than just the symptoms of your issues. Your body is constantly changing, and your health strategies should follow suit.

If you would like more information or some tips on common issues that we help with, please visit our web pages below. You'll have the option to download a free report that I created for you.

Back Pain: www.nextlevelpthouston.com/back-pain

Neck Pain: www.nextlevelpthouston.com/neck-pain

Shoulder Pain: www.nextlevelpthouston.com/shoulder-pain

Knee Pain: www.nextlevelpthouston.com/knee-pain

Hip and Sciatica Pain: www.nextlevelpthouston.com/hip-sciatica-pain

Foot/Ankle Pain: www.nextlevelpthouston.com/foot-ankle-pain

If you can't access the links above, you can always get the reports through our main page: www.nextlevelpthouston.com

You can also call our office at **281-888-0047** to request a copy of one of our reports. If you are feeling stuck and would like to speak to a specialist about your health-related issue, you can schedule a free, 20-minute phone call with one of our physical therapists.

To claim the free phone consultation, visit our website at www.nextlevelpthouston.com/phone-request and fill out the 1 minute survey. Or call my office at **281-888-0047**. I look forward to speaking with you.

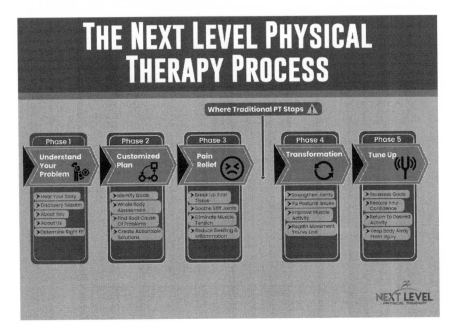

IF NOTHING CHANGES, NOTHING CHANGES

While I like to believe that every person reading this book will take the necessary steps to transform their health, I also know that some require more guidance and accountability to reach their goals. Knowledge is not power unless you implement it. In order for you to change your health, you have to change your mindset, physical activity, environment, nutrition, and stress management. Adversity is your friend. Take small, consistent steps to implement changes into your lifestyle and you will see significant benefits.

I want to thank you for supporting me in bringing more awareness to the public on ways to live healthy and thrive using natural solutions. It all starts with awareness that there is a problem. This will lead to clarity on which actions you can take. When you focus on the right actions, you will get positive results. When positive results compound over time, you get momentum.

If you found this book helpful, please pass it along to someone who might benefit. We are committed to helping everyone get unstuck from their health-related problems, so feel free to contact us to chat, wherever you are on your health journey.

www.nextlevelpthouston.com

REFERENCES

Bogduk, Nikolai. "Management of chronic low back pain." *Medical journal of Australia* 180.2 (2004): 79-83.

Levy, Becca R., Martin D. Slade, and Stanislav V. Kasl. "Longitudinal benefit of positive self-perceptions of aging on functional health." *The Journals of Gerontology Series B: Psychological Sciences and Social Sciences* 57.5 (2002): P409-P417.

Johannes, Catherine B., et al. "The prevalence of chronic pain in United States adults: results of an Internet-based survey." *The Journal of Pain* 11.11 (2010): 1230-1239.

Nourbakhsh, Mohammad Reza, and Amir Massoud Arab. "Relationship between mechanical factors and incidence of low back pain." *Journal of Orthopaedic & Sports Physical Therapy* 32.9 (2002): 447-460.

Katz, Jeffrey N., et al. "Surgery versus physical therapy for a meniscal tear and osteoarthritis." *New England Journal of Medicine* 368.18 (2013): 1675-1684.

Sihvonen, Raine, et al. "Arthroscopic partial meniscectomy versus sham surgery for a degenerative meniscal tear." *New England Journal of Medicine* 369.26 (2013): 2515-2524.

Tempelhof, Siegbert, Stefan Rupp, and Romain Seil. "Age-related prevalence of rotator cuff tears in asymptomatic shoulders." *Journal of shoulder and elbow surgery* 8.4 (1999): 296-299.

Giugliano, Dario, Antonio Ceriello, and Katherine Esposito. "The effects of diet on inflammation: emphasis on the metabolic syndrome." *Journal of the American College of Cardiology* 48.4 (2006): 677-685.

Grossman, Paul, et al. "Mindfulness-based stress reduction and health benefits: A meta-analysis." *Journal of psychosomatic research* 57.1 (2004): 35-43.

Lally, Phillippa, et al. "How are habits formed: Modelling habit formation in the real world." *European journal of social psychology* 40.6 (2010): 998-1009.

Warburton, Darren ER, Crystal Whitney Nicol, and Shannon SD Bredin. "Health benefits of physical activity: the evidence." *Cmaj* 174.6 (2006): 801-809.

Health Disclaimer

We make every effort to ensure that we accurately represent the injury advice and prognosis displayed throughout this book. However, examples of injuries and their prognosis are based on typical representations of those injuries that we commonly see in our physical therapy clinic. The information given is not intended as representations of every individual's potential injury.

As with any injury, each person's symptoms can vary widely and each person's recovery from injury can also vary depending upon background, genetics, previous medical history, application of exercises, posture, motivation to follow physical therapist's advice and various other physical factors. It is impossible to give a 100% complete accurate diagnosis and prognosis without a thorough physical examination and likewise the advice given for management of an injury cannot be deemed fully accurate in the absence of this examination from one of the physical therapists at Next Level Physical Therapy INC.

Significant injury risk is possible if you do not follow due diligence and seek suitable professional advice about your injury. No guarantees of specific results are expressly made or implied in this book.